Mindful Wellness

The Art of Sustained Weight Loss

by

Mack Fernsby

Mindful Wellness:

The Art of Sustained Weight Loss

Table of Contents

Introduction:
Embracing a Mindful Wellness Journey

Commencing a journey towards wellness is akin to embarking on a voyage of self-discovery, where each step taken is integral to the forging of a healthier, more vibrant self. With contemplative consideration, we lace up our proverbial walking shoes for an odyssey that encompasses the body, the mind, and the very spirit in which we endeavor to thrive. In this introductory traverse, we shall be delving into the essence of what it truly means to embrace a mindful wellness journey.

Wellness, a term amply used yet often misunderstood, is to be perceived as more than the mere absence of illness or ailment. It is the proactive pursuit of a lifestyle in balance: a symphony of nutrition, exercise, sleep, and emotional equilibrium. Engage with me, as we discover the joys of nurturing our physical vessels with the very sustenance that keeps us vital and vigorous. Let's explore the contours and rhythms of movement, imparting to our bodies the strength and flexibility they desire.

Imagine an approach to wellness that is painted with the broad strokes of conscious decision-making and insights. Your body, a canvas, is awaiting your hand to blend the colors of healthy eating habits and considered physical activity into a masterpiece of personal well-being. Allow each flourish of the brush to be guided by an awareness of the present moment—moment to moment, bite by bite, and stretch by stretch.

Wellness is a journey marked by its undulating terrain. At the crux of this odyssey lies the psychology of eating—a complex interplay between our emotional landscape and the choices we make at the dining table. Here, we shall not venture deep into strategies for hunger mindfulness or emotional eating; rather, let this serve as an invocation for the profound reflections to follow in the subsequent chapters.

As we chart the course of this journey, understand that wellness is not a universal prescription but an intimate conversation with one's own body and soul. What resonates harmony for one may not echo the same for another, and thus, the map we draw will be one of personalization, inked with our unique aspirations and intentions.

The path to a healthier self is not linear. It spirals, plateaus, and at times, seems to march in place. We'll sketch out the contour lines of these plateaus later on, but it's within these moments of seeming stagnation that a steadfast spirit is cultivated, a spirit acquainted with patience and perseverance.

Stress, that silent saboteur of serenity and wellness, shall inevitably weave its way into our lives as we progress along this path. A segment of our journey must be allocated to gaining mastery over this unwelcome visitor, harnessing mindfulness techniques to disentangle ourselves from its clutches.

Let us not forget the vital role of exercise in this grand scheme of health. The act of movement can transform into a meditative mantra for the mind, a component that will later be unveiled in its full texture and color. Think of it not merely as a box to be checked but as a rhythm to be felt, a flow to be found.

Our nutritional compass will point us towards an equilibrium—harmony between carbs, proteins, and the often-misunderstood fats—illustrating the concept of macronutrient mastery and the inadvertent power harbored by the greenest of greens. But again, let's not overindulge in these morsels of insight just yet.

On this passage, no traveler is an island. We thrive in togetherness, building tribes and seeking expertise when our own lanterns flicker and dim. The support system we establish can be the difference between faltering steps and a bold stride forwards.

Self-compassion is a treasure along this road, a gentle reminder to favor progress over impractical quests for perfection. This journey is festooned with milestones to be celebrated, each one a testament to the strength and dedication harbored within. We shall lift our cups to each success and, in doing so, fortify ourselves for the continued adventure ahead.

Underpinning our wellness journey is the science of metabolism—a dynamic engine of our being that influences how we process the very fuel we consume. It is not static but evolves as we age, and we shall touch upon its mysteries and management throughout these pages.

Should you find your well of motivation drying or your progress impeded by unseen hurdles, we will delve into the methods to maintain your drive and navigate around obstacles. Visualization, affirmations, and a collection of practical tactics – these are the tools that shall secure your footing on this hike towards health.

As foretold, our journey shall incorporate integrative approaches to weight loss, inviting holistic practices to partake in our quest for wellness, and even take a closer look at the supportive role vitamins and minerals can play when summoned wisely.

In these opening remarks, let us attune ourselves to the concept of a mindful wellness journey. A sojourn that transcends mere physical transformation and weaves into the fabric of our daily existence. Our expedition commences, not at the start line of a race but on the threshold of an awakening—a recognition of the interconnectedness of body, mind, and the world we inhabit.

Together, let us step forward with intent and curiosity, our eyes fixed not just on the horizon but on every petal, pebble, and pattern that adorns our path. To a journey where each step is a dance, a mindful step towards a fuller, richer, and more wondrous life.

Chapter 1:
The Wellness Wheel: Understanding the Components

In this grand unfolding of our journey toward health and wellness, we turn to the essence of our quest: The Wellness Wheel. A compass for those who seek to navigate the seas of a balanced life, each spoke of this wheel represents a crucial aspect of well-being, and all must turn in harmony for the voyage to be smooth. **Nutrition** forms the foundation, where we indulge not only in the pleasures of taste but also in the fortitude of mindful nourishment. **Exercise**, that lively dance of movement, fortifies our bodies and hearts, each beat a drum propelling us onward—be it through the vitality of cardiovascular health, the might of strength training, or the grace of cultivating flexibility. And let's not forget the serene oasis of **sleep**, without which no journey can sustain; it is the restorative silence that whispers secrets of weight management in our ears. Here in Chapter 1, let's unravel the intricate tapestry of these elements, understanding them not in isolation, but as integrated threads woven into the fabric of our being—each a color, each a texture contributing to the masterpiece of personal wellness. Indeed, to grasp the Wheel in its entirety is to embrace the very art of living.

Nutrition: Eating for a Mindful Body

In this tableau of our lives, amidst the vivid strokes of daily hustle and flow, what we consume plays the leading role for a grand performance. The art of eating extends beyond the mere satiation of hunger; it's a meditative ritual for the mindful body. Picture, if you will, the nutrients as paint on an artist's palette—a spectrum of colors to adorn the canvas of our well-being.

One might ask, "What does it mean to eat mindfully?" It's a dance of savoring flavors while being acutely aware of the body's needs, the source of food, and its effects on both our physical and mental states. To eat with intention is to choose foods that elevate our health, instead of those that merely tantalize our taste buds with fleeting joy.

Imagine a meal as a symphony, with each ingredient contributing its unique note to the harmony of nutrition. In the absence of processed foods filled with additives, our bodies begin to revel in the wholesomeness of natural, unrefined choices. Grains that haven't been stripped of their fiber sing melodies of sustained energy. Lean proteins lend their rhythm, repairing and building our tissues, while vegetables and fruits, those vibrant virtuosos, impart antioxidants to reduce the cacophony of inflammation.

Consumption is an ongoing discovery, a lesson in the balance of macronutrients and the whisper-soft footsteps of micronutrients as they bolster our bodily functions. Eating a variety of foods ensures we conduct the full orchestra of vitamins and minerals necessary for optimal health.

Hydration, the unsung hero of our physiological tale, must not be overlooked. Every cell in our body yearns for water—it is the elixir of life, the fluidity in our movement, the clarity in our thoughts. A well-hydrated body is akin to a bubbling stream, full of vigor and life, whereas dehydration leaves us as parched as a withered leaf at summer's end.

Let's not forget the aspect of timing when it comes to feasting. Listening to our body's natural cues and eating at regular intervals can prevent the all-too-common extreme hunger that leads to overindulgence. When our body languishes too long without sustenance, the sudden bounty of a meal can be devoured mindlessly, leaving us bloated on the shores of regret.

The notion of portion control is another aspect where mindfulness takes center stage. It's not merely about reducing quantities but understanding appropriate serving sizes that maintain harmony in our system. Sensible portions can be less enthralling than the lure of an overflowing plate, yet their subtlety is key to maintaining a balanced composition.

Navigating the sea of dietary trends can bewilder the bravest of souls. Yet, adhering to a diet simply because it's in vogue is akin to wearing someone else's shoes and expecting to comfortably walk a mile. Each body is its own unique landscape, with hills and valleys that may require different sustenance than what's popular.

To eat mindfully is to engage in the profound intimacy of knowing one's body, learning how food influences energy levels, moods, and overall vitality. It's a personal journey where one discovers not only the joy of flavors but the lasting contentment of health.

Snacking, often vilified as the sly saboteur of wellness, can in fact be part of a mindful eating strategy. Healthy snacks can act as bridges between meals, preventing the dips in energy and mood that might cause one to seek refuge in less nourishing options. These pit stops, when stocked with nutritious choices, keep the motor of our metabolism humming with finesse.

Within this sphere, it's crucial to recognize the role of indulgence. To deny oneself the pleasure of an occasional treat is to walk a tightrope without a safety net. A mindful approach allows pleasures in moderation, savored without guilt, as part of the spectrum of eating that nourishes both body and soul.

Consciously navigating the social aspect of eating is equally important. Meals shared with others can bring joy and connection, yet peer pressure to eat certain foods or to overeat can stir turbulence in the waters. Standing at the helm, with a clear sense of our nutritional course, allows us to partake in social feasting without being swept away by the current.

In the journey of mindful eating, the exploration of foods from diverse cultures can be an odyssey of discovery. Exotic spices and unheard-of grains expand our culinary horizons, introducing not only new tastes but also varied nutrients that enrich our eating repertoire.

As we continue through the chapters of our wellness wheel, let us carry with us the thread of mindfulness in nutrition, weaving it into the very fabric of our being. Engage with your meals as one would a cherished friend—listen intently, savor the presence, and honor the nourishment it provides.

The act of eating, when done with reverence, becomes more than ingestion—it transforms into a pilgrimage towards health and tranquility, a profound ritual where every bite is a step on the path of well-being. And thus, with mindful choices on our fork, we sculpt the temple of our bodies with care and wisdom, culminating in a masterpiece that is as much about exquisite taste as it is about exquisite health.

Exercise: Moving for a Healthier Self

Amidst the grand tapestry of wellness, the act of exercise stands as a vibrant thread, weaving strength and vitality into the very fabric of our being. Within the realm of the Wellness Wheel, movement is akin to a dynamic symphony, where every stretch, lift, and stride contributes to the profound masterpiece of a healthier self. Delving into the heart of this section, we eschew the detail of cardiovascular peaks and strength training intricacies, instead focusing on the invigorating essence of exercise. By embracing physical activity, we not only sculpt a more resilient body but also ignite the flames of mental clarity and emotional balance, propelling us forward on our quest for weight loss and fitness milestones. Let's not just move, but move with intention and joy, embracing the richness of activity that can transform daily existence into a dance of wellness that echoes with each pulse and breath.

Cardiovascular Health: The Heart of Fitness

In the rhythmic echoes of our heartbeat, there lies a tale as old as time, the saga of life itself. As we shift our gaze within to explore the effervescent dance of cardiorespiratory fitness, let's entwine our understanding around the vital importance it holds in our quest for wellness. The heart, my friends, is not merely an organ. It's the engine of our vitality; the very drum that beats the rhythm of our existence.

In days of yore, the sages understood that a strong heart was paramount for an invigorating life. This truth endures - now, backed by the hard evidence of science. For those seeking weight loss, fitness, and mental health improvements, neglect not your cardiovascular health, for it is the cornerstone of your temple, the body.

Let us conceive of the cardiovascular system as a network of roads. When well-maintained, travel (or blood flow) is unimpeded; commerce (or nutrient and oxygen exchange) flourishes. A sedentary lifestyle, though, is akin to the slow build-up of traffic, obstructions that lead to complications and harm the heart's efficiency.

To engage in cardiovascular exercise, then, is to clear these roads, strengthen the cardiac muscle, and improve the body's ability to use oxygen. Aerobic activities like brisk walking, cycling, swimming, and running, elevate the heart rate, teaching the mighty muscle to pump more effectively both at work and at rest.

As one delves into this art of fitness, it's essential to tailor one's endeavors to the whisperings of the heart. Begin gently, with activities that quicken the pulse but allow for conversation. Over time, as a blacksmith tempers steel, so must you temper your heart with incrementally more challenging exercises.

An equilibrium between exertion and rest must be struck, as well. Just as the waves caress the shore with might, then retreat softly, giving the sand reprieve, so too must we alternate high intensity with adequate rest. Adhering to a well-crafted exercise plan not only bolsters heart health but fortifies the soul, invigorating the lifeblood of our spirit.

Moreover, let's not overlook the interplay between heart function and weight. A healthy cardiovascular system plays a significant role in metabolism and the body's ability to shed excess pounds. A vibrant heart hums like a bird in flight, swiftly, elegantly, optimizing the combustion of calories throughout the day.

As the heart grows stronger, so does its alliance with the lungs. This dynamic duo, enhanced through regular cardio, improves the tenacity of one's entire being, propelling the practitioner towards peaks previously unattainable, through forests of doubt, and into clearings of self-discovery.

The benefits extend beyond the corporeal, into the realm of the mind. A healthy, robust cardiovascular system can act as a sentinel against stress, anxiety, and the blue moods that occasionally cloud our horizons. With every thud of the heart, myriad hormones cascade, some that soothe the tempests within, affording moments of blissful peace amidst the tumult of life.

It's momentous, too, that as we till the soil of fitness, we prepare our bodies for the advancing years. A well-tuned cardiovascular system may fend off the ravages of time, ensuring that the twilight years are illuminated with vigor rather than dimmed by fatigue.

One mustn't overlook the power of consistency. As the sun rises each day with reliable splendor, so must we rise to the challenge of nurturing our heart's health with daily practices. Consistent cardiovascular exercise transforms the transient into the eternal – the fleeting moments of effort coalesce into enduring strength.

And what of those embarking on this journey amidst the chaos of life's many burdens? Fear not, for the commitment to cardiovascular health need not be onerous. Even the busiest of bees can find pockets of time to stretch their wings, to flutter and fly in the vast skies of physical activity.

Finding the balance between life's demands and the siren call of wellness can indeed seem a Herculean task. Yet, remember, amidst every challenge lies opportunity; in every drop of sweat, a chance for renewal. The pursuit of cardiovascular health, therefore, is not merely a physical endeavor. It's a pledge to oneself, a sacred vow to honor the body's needs and the heart's whispers.

Finally, let's acknowledge the journey's inherent ebb and flow. There may be setbacks, times when the heart feels heavy and the path to wellness steep. But through dedication and an unyielding spirit, these moments can be transformed into stepping stones towards greater health and happiness.

And so, with the drum of our heartbeat as our guide, we march forward in the pursuit of fitness, hand in hand with the knowledge that at the core of our health resides a powerful truth: A hearty, boundless, vivacious cardiovascular system is not just the heart of fitness – it's the very essence of a life well-lived.

Strength Training: Building a Resilient Body

In the grand tapestry of fitness, the warp threads that provide its strength and structure are made of robust strands known as strength training. It's where sinew and bone grow resistant to the ravages of time, where muscles extol their power, and where the very sinews of our resilience are fortified. Yes, to stroll on the path of wellness is to embrace not only the whispering flow of a gentle yoga stretch but also the resolute clang of the iron weights that challenge our physical being.

Now, one might inquire, why place such an emphasis on the rigorous endeavors of strength training in the pursuit of health and wellness? The answer, succinct though it may be, is that building muscle is akin to weaving armor around one's body; an armor against injury, against disease, and against the decline that time so eagerly plots. And it is not merely the bodybuilder or the athlete who stands to benefit, but every individual yearning for vitality.

Commence with the understanding that muscles are metabolic furnaces, glowing with the fire that consumes calories. With each additional pound of muscle, your body burns more calories, even whilst you are nestled in repose. This is a wondrous ally in the quest for weight management, as it aids in tipping the delicate scales of energy balance in favor of leanness.

But let us delve deeper. The might of one's muscles is critical in maintaining independence as the years accumulate like pages in a ponderous tome. With strength comes the ability to perform the ballet of daily activities with grace – be it carrying groceries, bounding up a flight of stairs, or ensconcing oneself in the comforting embrace of an armchair without calling upon assistance.

To foster the growth of strength requires an engagement with resistance. This resistance can come from the heft of an iron dumbbell, the tension of a rubber band, or even the weight of one's own body enacted against gravity's relentless pull. The key lies in subjecting the muscles to a challenge, coaxing them into becoming more potent than they were the day prior.

There is a rhythmic beauty to the progression of strength training. One begins tentatively, perhaps, with weights that seem to scoff at their feeble attempt to lift them. Yet, consistency proves to be a most loyal companion. Over time, what was once a trial becomes a triumph, as heavier weights rise in a testament to newly forged power.

In crafting a regimen of strength training, diversity is the jewel in its crown. Engaging different muscle groups not only sculpts the physique but ensures that all components of our musculature sing in harmony. A symphony of squats, lunges, presses, and pulls that allows us to be both the composer and the conductor of our physical destiny.

An often overlooked character in this narrative of strength is the rest period. It is during this interlude, amidst the quieting of clattering weights, that muscles find rejuvenation. Without rest, there is no repair, and without repair, there is no growth. Therefore, it is imperative to weave in days of respite between the days of vigor.

Let us also speak of technique, for technique is the artist's brushstroke on the canvas. Proper form is a whisper of safety to the joints, a promise of efficacy to the muscles, a mantra of longevity for the body. To lift incorrectly is to invite dissent from our corporeal form, to cultivate risk where there should be reward.

Within strength training, there resides the potential for transformation not only of the body but also of the mind. As the body conquers new frontiers of strength, so too does the mind fortify its own resolve. The discipline of lifting heavier, the perseverance in facing formidable resistance, these are the crucibles where mental robustness is honed.

Now, while some may pursue strength training within the hallowed halls of a gym, others might choose the sanctuary of their home – for strength does not demand an audience. Whether it takes root amidst the symphony of weights and machines or in the quietude of a living room, the growth of muscle is indifferent to location.

Nutrition, while not the central star in this discussion, remains an indispensable understudy to strength training. It is the sustenance that feeds the muscles, the fuel that powers the furnace. An alliance between exercise and eating, between protein and plyometrics, is where the alchemy of true transformation lies.

As we continue our journey through the wellness wheel, from nutrition to exercise, let us carry with us the knowledge that strength training is not an esoteric rite reserved for the mighty. It is, instead, a universal prescription for durability, a legacy of vitality that we can bestow upon ourselves regardless of age or station.

The caliber of our lives is dictated not by the turning of years, but by the strength we harbor within. To embrace strength training is to embrace a resoluteness that can weather the storms of time. It is a pact we make—a covenant with ourselves—to build a body that is not merely a vessel, but a resilient citadel.

And so, we come to understand that strength training is not merely a facet of physicality; it is a beacon that guides us towards a haven of health and wellness. It carves out a form not just impressive in aesthetics, but formidable in function. Let us then lift, and in lifting, ascend to the greater heights of our human potential.

Flexibility: Cultivating a Supple Structure As we embark further into the journey of wellness, with nutrition and various forms of exercise already woven into the tapestry of our routine, let's now delve into the realm of flexibility - a vital yet often overlooked aspect of health and fitness. Flexibility, the very essence of adaptability and grace, speaks volumes in the pursuit of a body and mind in harmonious alignment.

The art of stretching is as old as the hills, with ancient roots and modern relevance. Consider for a moment the grace of a dancer, the ease of a cat stretching in the sun, or even the instinctive morning stretch that unfurls your body upon waking. These images evoke a sense of freedom and a whisper of potential; and this very suppleness is within your reach.

Why then, you might ponder, is flexibility so pivotal? Our muscles, all too often constrained by the shackles of sedentary lifestyles and the tyranny of the chair, cry out for movement. The fibers within them can become shortened, tight, and ultimately lead to discomfort, pain, and a susceptibility to injury. Stretching, therefore, becomes a liberating force for our musculature.

Flexibility doesn't merely confer physical benefits. When you imbue your structure with the leniency of well-stretched muscles, you're also greasing the cogs of your mental machinery. Stress, that gnarly beast that often accompanies our daily endeavors, has a tendency to lodge itself in our physical frames. A solid stretching regimen can be the very elixir to this bodily tension.

As for the novice aspirants to flexibility, fear not, for starting is as simple as reaching for your toes or pulling an arm across your chest. The beauty of this practice lies in its accessibility; there's no requirement for elaborate apparatus or a hefty membership fee. Stretching can be integrated seamlessly into your daily life, whether it be through yoga, a post-workout routine, or even discreet office desk stretches.

For those with their eyes set on shedding weight and sculpting a physique, flexibility is a crucial ally. A flexible body is one that moves more efficiently, thus enabling more effective workouts and reducing the chance of exercise-related injuries that could derail your progress.

It is important to note that like any worthwhile endeavor, the path to flexibility does not run straight, nor does it abide by the fallacy of instant gratification. It demands consistency and patience, as the increments of improvement are often gradual. The celebration, though, lies in the journey rather than the destination, with each stride towards flexibility offering a little more ease in the physical narrative you live out each day.

Consider, if you will, a life where bending to scoop up a child or reaching for that top shelf is not a source of strain but a simple, fluid motion. Flexibility can transform the mundane into the effortless, elevating your standard of living in subtle yet profound ways.

Some might inquire about the ideal frequency of stretching, to which I propose a daily rendezvous with your suppler self. Incorporate it into your morning arousal from sleep or as a tranquil epilogue to your day. If daily proves too ambitious, start where you are able; for each moment spent in the pursuit of flexibility is an investment in your corporeal treasury.

Let's not forget that flexibility is not a lone soldier but part of an integral battalion of wellness. It complements the strength built through resistance training and the stamina gained from cardiovascular efforts. These three share an intertwined fate, each enhancing the effectiveness of the other.

To those embedded in the rigorous pursuit of fitness, flexibility offers a nurturing respite for the muscles tasked with the heavy lifting and the heart charged with pumping vitality. Here, in the quietude of stretching, is where recovery weaves its restorative magic.

There's an inclusivity to flexibility that beckons to all corners of humanity. Young or old, embroiled in fitness or new to the motion, the invitation to stretch is universally extended. There are stretches tailored for every age, every body type, and every level of fitness. It's not about performing acrobatic feats but about personal betterment and the daily quest for an enriched quality of life.

In this supple pursuit, there are tools at your disposal, should you opt to utilize them. The foam roller - a cylinder of salvation for sore muscles, the resistance band - an ally in amplifying the stretch, and the stability ball - a partner in enhancing balance and flexibility. All these serve as adjuncts to your efforts, bolstering your stretch regimen.

Embarking on the quest towards a more flexible self also brings with it lessons of humility. One must recognize the current limitations and appreciate that the body has boundaries that demand respect. To stretch with ego is to invite injury; to stretch with mindfulness is to embrace growth.

In sum, the cultivation of a supple structure is more than a mere mechanical endeavor. It's a narrative that unfolds with each elongation of your muscles. It's a dialogue between your body and mind, each stretch a stanza in the poem of your well-being. Embrace flexibility, and you unfurl not only your body but the very horizons of your healthful pursuit.

Sleep: Restorative Practices for Weight Management

Slumber, often underestimated, wields a powerful force in the intricate dance of weight management. In the symphony of wellness where each component plays a critical role, sleep emerges as the restorative pause, often glossed over in the rush of our daily lives but crucial to the balance sought by those endeavoring to shape their wellbeing.

Amidst the quest for vitality through nutrition and exercise, many embark on journeys that neglect the silent healer of night. Sleep rejuvenates the weary muscles and the taxed mind, granting reprieve that nourishes more than mere energy levels. Here, in the soft embrace of rest, the body conducts its covert symphony—repairing tissues, harmonizing hormones, and finessing metabolic functions that are imperative to weight management.

Research unveils that sleep quality and quantity intimately converse with our waistlines. The lack thereof intensifies cravings and muddles the brain's ability to make judicious food choices. It's akin to sailing through a storm on turbulent seas, where persistent sleep deprivation leaves one vulnerable to the sirens of sugar and fat.

Dive into the restorative embrace of sleep, and you'll discover that a consistent, quality rest can serve as your ally against reactionary eating. It's an invigorating cycle, as enhanced energy levels spurned by restful nights fuel workouts, bolstering the fortitude needed to resist temptation's call. Let this be your nocturnal haven—a place where recovery underpins the hard-earned victories of daytime discipline.

Consider those nights when sleep eludes, wrangling you into hours of restless tossing. The dawn often greets not with fresh perspective but with a body in inadvertent rebellion, sluggish metabolism dragging in its wake. In these dawns without proper rest, hormones like ghrelin and leptin—our hunger conductors—fall out of tune, playing discordant notes that bewitch our sense of satiety and hunger.

To achieve serene slumber's equilibrium, we must heed the setting. Envision your sleeping chamber as a sanctuary, where soothing hues and tranquil silence court the whispers of sleep. The mattress, a cozy altar; the room, a temple stripped of electronic distractions, where the air, lightly perfumed with lavender or chamomile, lulls and mends the spirit.

And when night's curtain falls, routine is the steady rhythm that beckons sleep forth. A calming prelude—a book or meditation—replaces the frantic tempo of screens and their blue light crescendos which jar the senses and postpone rest's arrival. Your moments before sleep are a ritual to be refined, where calming practices are invitations to a restorative respite.

For within the hush of night, the stillness belies a world in flux—a body in delicate conversation with itself. Hormones cascade, orchestrating dreams and regulating appetite while cells renew and repair. Here, ghrelin's call is tempered, leptin's satisfaction found, and insulin sensitivity honed, all steeped in the silent symphony of sleep.

Consider the night watchman, whose irregular shifts pirate away consistent sleep cycles. Their plight reveals that it's not merely sleep, but its rhythmic regularity that is a stalwart guardian of metabolic health. Thus, adhere to a schedule as one would a sacred script, letting your internal clock set a metronomic cadence for your slumbers.

For those navigating the seas of sleeplessness, be not dissuaded by transient tumult. Strategies abound for the weary sailor adrift—breathing exercises that billow the sails of relaxation, visualizations that chart courses through turbulent thoughts, and perhaps a mindful sip of warm, calming tea to course through you like a balm.

In the voyage of weight management, heed the nuggets of wisdom derived from time's enduring passage—where feasts encroach upon slumber's domain only to stoke the embers of indigestion that keep rest at bay and entice discomfort to linger like a vigilant specter at the bedside.

Too, let us not dismiss the gentle exertion that precedes our descent into the night's embrace—a soothing stroll beneath the stars, where the mind unfurls and the day's stresses dissolve like mist into the ether, paving the way for a peaceful surrender to the sandman's tender clasp.

Thus equipped with the know-how of sleep's paramount role in weight management, let us champion our nocturnal journeys as ardently as we do the daytime pursuit of health and vitality. For in the delicate balance of the wellness wheel, sleep is the oft-forgotten cogs and gears, flawlessly operating beneath the surface to maintain the machine's relentless motion towards equilibrium and health.

Now, as you adjourn from this ode to rest's powerful sway, consider how tonight, as every night, you will lay the groundwork for tomorrow's wellness. Let sleep become your trusted companion on this journey, an unwavering ally, a restorative force to be woven into the fabric of your daily life, as indispensable as the air we breathe and the sustenance we consume. Embrace its silken threads and weave a tapestry of health, resplendent and robust, in the grand design of your wellness story.

Chapter 2:
The Psychology of Eating

Embarking on the wellness odyssey, one might easily forget that the battlefield of health is not just forged of which leafy greens to embrace or what shiny new exercise regimen sparkles with promise, but also the intricate, whispered conversations within the convoluted chambers of our minds. The voyage from awareness to change cruises through the serpentine river of our psychological relationship with food. We often sail these waters unaware of how the riptides of emotion tug at our eating habits, drawing us to feast in the absence of hunger. To truly set a course for lasting wellbeing and a svelte waist, one must become an astute listener of the body's murmurs, teasing apart the tangled strands of physiological need from emotional yearning. In this crucible of transformation, we're not simply seeking ephemeral success, but the crafting of sustainable habits, tempered in the smithy of mindful consistency. This profound journey into the psychology of eating isn't a mere chapter; it's the compass by which we navigate the deeper waters of health, fitness, and mental tranquility—the sanctum where our nourishment choices become allies in the noble quest for wellness.

Emotional Eating: Navigating Food and Feelings

The interweaving tapestry of our emotions and food choices forms a complex narrative that far exceeds the simple act of eating for sustenance. Emotional eating is a voyage through the tumultuous sea of our sentiments, where many find themselves reaching for the helm in the form of a chocolate bar or a bag of chips. Why do these edible items become so entwined with our feelings? How can we steer the ship towards healthier horizons?

At the heart of emotional eating lies a paradox; food becomes both our comforter and our captor. In moments of sadness, stress, or even boredom, we are often drawn to food for its promise of immediate pleasure. Yet, the solace provided by such indulgences is fleeting, and we're soon left with the aftertaste of guilt or the weight of physical discomfort.

It's essential to acknowledge that emotional eating is not a mere lack of willpower. It is an intricate ballet of physiological cues, psychological coping mechanisms, and societal signals. Our brains are wired to associate certain foods, usually high in sugar, fat, or both, with reward and relief. Thus, a cycle is born, one in which we seek out these foods to self-soothe, only to perpetuate an unending dance.

To illuminate this subject further, consider the alchemy of a stressful day. As tension weaves itself into the fabric of our being, the body's hormones, namely cortisol, reach out for help. High-calorie, sugary or fatty foods tend to provide an antidote, albeit temporary, to calm the storm inside. This biological response is rooted in survival mechanisms, but it direly misinterprets the stress of modern life as a signal to stockpile energy.

Understanding these underpinnings, however, is only half the battle. To navigate emotional eating, one must also foster self-awareness. Pause and ponder, are you truly hungry, or is there an emotional undertow tugging at your appetite? Teasing apart physical hunger from emotional hunger is a skill, one that requires attentiveness and mindfulness.

When the whisper of emotional hunger murmurs, it's crucial to listen carefully but not surrender to impulse. Distraction can be a powerful ally. Engage in an activity you enjoy, something that occupies both mind and body. Perhaps a walk outside, where nature's embrace offers its own kind of comfort, far removed from the clutches of the pantry.

Another beacon in the fog of emotional eating is communication. Vocalizing our struggles, fears, and frustrations to a compassionate listener can alleviate the need to channel these emotions through food. In conversation, our feelings become externalized, diminishing their power to drive us towards emotional eating.

As we cultivate healthier responses to our emotions, it's equally important to stock our kitchens mindfully. If temptation is within easy reach, the journey to healthy eating habits will be fraught with peril. Instead, surround yourself with nourishing options that support your wellness goals. Even in times of emotional tumult, you'll find comfort in knowing the choices at hand are kinder to your body.

An indispensable part of this navigation is self-forgiveness. To falter is human, and indulging in response to emotions doesn't mark failure. It presents an opportunity to learn, to understand your triggers better, and to plan a more resilient strategy for the future.

Food, imbued with the power of tradition and collective memory, shouldn't become an adversary. It's possible to celebrate food and respect its place in our lives without letting it cloud our emotions. A slice of birthday cake is a slice of joy, not guilt, when consumed with presence and appreciation.

Lest we forget, the company we keep at the table can nourish us as much as the meal itself. Sharing meals with friends or family can act as an anchoring ritual, a time to slow down, to engage, and to relish the communal aspect of eating. Here, food becomes a medium for connection, not a tool for emotional escape.

For those traversing particularly troublesome terrain in their relationship with food and feelings, professional guidance may be the lighthouse that steers them from the rocky shores. Dietitians, therapists, and wellness coaches offer expertise in navigating these waters, providing support, accountability, and coping strategies tailored to individual needs.

It is also prudent to emphasize the importance of routine. Regular, balanced meals create a rhythm for our bodies, helping to stabilize mood and energy levels. When we're nourished and satisfied, the siren song of emotional eating loses its allure, and we're better equipped to weather the emotional storms.

The path through emotional eating is not linear; it winds and loops, offering lessons with each turn. As you embark on this journey, patience and persistence are your companions, reminding you that each day presents a new chance to align your food choices with your wellness vision. And through the process, you'll cultivate not just a healthier eating pattern, but also a profound understanding of yourself, one bite at a time.

In the realm of emotional eating, recall that food is meant to sustain and delight us, not to serve as a crutch for our emotions. It's a balance of nourishment and enjoyment, an equilibrium that supports both the body and the spirit. As we close the chapter on emotional eating, bear in mind the facets of food that bring us together, that celebrate our humanity, and that offer joy without eclipsing our wellness.

Hunger Mindfulness: Listening to Your Body

Hunger is a primordial signal, a dance of exquisite complexity that speaks of needs, desires, and the very essence of survival. In the realm of wellness, we often overlook this subtle conversation, opting instead for strict regimens and external cues to dictate when and what we should eat. Yet, in the ebb and flow of daily life, there lies a profound truth waiting to be uncovered—it's the language of your body, a language that cries out to be spoken and understood through hunger mindfulness.

Embarking on this path, it's essential to unravel the tapestry of signals that your body sends. There's a distinction as clear as night from day between true physical hunger and the emotional pangs that masquerade as a need to eat. To become attuned to your body's hunger cues is to step into a world where each rumble and pang is a message, a directive from the body's innate wisdom guiding you toward nourishment.

Listening begins with silence, a pause in the incessant bustle of life. When hunger whispers or shouts, take a moment to inquire within. Is it the hollow feeling of an empty stomach, the slight dizziness of depleted energy stores that beckons you to the table? Or are you seeking solace, comfort, or distraction in the sweet embrace of food? Hunger mindfulness requires that you become a detective of your own experience, questioning and discovering with each hunger call.

Consider the rhythms of your meals, a vital component in this listening exercise. Society often pushes the narrative of three squares a day—a framework that can both support and confound. Your body's truths are unique and may not fit into these prescribed time slots. Be mindful of whether your eating habits align with your physiological needs or if they're merely a script you've been following without question.

Not every gnawing urge merits a meal or a snack. Thirst masquerades as hunger with cunning ease. At times, a glass of water is the elixir that the body truly craves, and your discernment between thirst and hunger becomes a powerful ally in your wellness journey. Take sips of clarity and become well-versed in the subtle distinctions. Hydration might just quell what seemed like a burgeoning hunger.

Mindfulness begets mastery, not in the sense of control, but as an art to be honed. You begin to recognize the spectrum of hunger—there are the shadows of a slight need, the contours of a moderate craving, and the bold strokes of urgent starvation. You learn not to let yourself waver to the extremes where choices become rash, and where wellness likely loses its foothold. Aim to address your needs before desperation takes the reins.

What of the food you choose when hunger resonates within you? It calls not only for quantity but also for quality. Let your body guide you to the selections it inherently knows are wholesome and satiating rather than to the transient pleasures of sugar-laden or highly processed temptations. Call upon the knowledge tucked away from previous chapters on nutrition, and stand firm against the siren songs that beckon you towards empty calories.

Mealtime is a sacred ceremony—a space and time that demand respect and presence. When you eat, do so with attention and intention. Fast-paced consumption blurs the lines of satiety and fullness. To dine mindfully is to taste each morsel, to chew thoroughly, to allow the food to settle, and to permit the signal of fullness to reach your mind before you consider seconds.

The act of tracking your hunger and its patterns over time is like planting seeds in a garden of self-awareness. Keep a log if you must, jotting down the instances of hunger, their severity, their true sources, and how you respond. Patterns will emerge, cycles will become apparent, and you will gain insights into how your physical activity, sleep quality, stress levels, and emotional states interweave with your cravings for sustenance.

Do not misjudge this practice as one of austerity or deprivation; rather, it's a celebration of attunement, of honoring what is needed. You may find that sometimes, the body craves more than food—it desires movement, rest, or connection. Listen deeply, and you might discover hidden hungers that feed not the stomach but the soul.

It's crucial, too, to forgive your lapses in mindfulness. There will be days when the chocolate calls louder than your wisdom, when comfort eating seems like the only balm to your storm. Recognize these moments, learn from them, and gently steer yourself back to the path of awareness without self-flagellation. Remember that every meal is a new opportunity to listen and to learn.

As part of our odyssey towards health and wellness, let us venture towards understanding the signals that our body relays to us—the beckoning for nourishment, the murmurings of preferences, and the loud declarations of deficits. You're not just feeding a body; you're nourishing a dynamic system in which every bite impacts your being's intricate web.

And when you do listen, when you truly hear what your body is saying and respond in kind, a transformation unfolds. You find that cravings hold less sway, that well-being isn't just a concept but a feeling—a sensation of lightness, of alignment, of being in sync with the body's own rhythms and needs.

This, my friends, is hunger mindfulness, the art and act of listening to your body. It's a chapter in a tale—no less enchanting for its science than for its soul—that's forever being written as you weave the strands of awareness into the tapestry of your everyday life. Practice it well, and the story of your wellness will be one of attunement, resonance, and a joyful harmony with the needs of your body.

Now, ready to delve deeper into the wellspring of knowledge, let us embark upon the journey of crafting sustainable habits, the next cornerstone in our exploration of the psychology of eating and the broader, richer narrative of true well-being.

Sustainable Habits: Creating Long-Term Success

In our search for wellbeing and control over the delicate art of eating, we find ourselves standing at the juncture of intention and habit. The psychology of eating is not simply a fleeting musing over the calories and the nutrients; it is, in fact, an intricate dance with our daily practices. So let us, then, delve into the cornerstones of sustainable habits that carve the path to long-term success.

Engrained within the tapestry of our routine, habits are the silent weavers of our day. Crafting a routine around mindful eating isn't a mere act of willpower; it is about building a structure that endures beyond the whims of momentary craving. We begin by setting the stage with small, but pivotal, choices that elevate our chance for lasting change. With each day's dawn, we can decide to start with a nutritious breakfast, setting our metabolic tempo.

Consider the power of repetition. As with a chorus repeated until the words are second nature, so our habits solidify with each iteration. To eat mindfully, then, we must cultivate repetition in our conscious choices until they become the familiar melody of our daily lives. The act of pausing before a meal to truly consider our hunger levels is one such practice. Repeat this enough, and it transforms from a conscious action into a reflexive assessment of need versus impulse.

As any worthy pursuit, there must be room for flexibility, for the unyielding tree snaps in a storm whilst the supple grasses bend and survive. Similarly, our habits must have the resilience to weather the buffet of unforeseen challenges. Should a certain routine no longer serve you, be it an ill-timed meal or a snack of lesser nutritional value, adjust it. Adapting to life's ever-changing tides helps maintain the course towards your wellness goals.

What of the company we keep, you might wonder. Indeed, surrounding oneself with fellow travelers on the journey towards mindful eating can offer both encouragement and accountability. Sharing meals with those who also revel in the slow savoring of each bite, who also discern the signals of satiety, can reinforce our own commitment to these practices.

Periodically, we must recalibrate and fine-tune our habits. This steady vigilance ensures they evolve in step with our lives. The milestone of progress, be it weight loss, improved fitness, or mental clarity, affords an opportunity to reflect. What habits have brought you thus far? What might need to be amended to carry you further on your journey?

Technology and resources available in our modern age can serve as an anchor for our habits. Tracking our food intake, planning our meals ahead of time, and having access to a plethora of healthy recipes at our fingertips can support our goals in maintaining a balanced diet and preventing overindulgence.

Consistency isn't about perfection; it's about progression. If you find yourself succumbing to an old pattern, it is not the time for self-reproach. Rather, it's a moment to understand the slip and reaffirm your commitment. Each day presents a new canvas upon which to illustrate your determination, painting over yesterday's blemishes with today's endeavors.

Many are tempted to rely on drastic measures—a sudden, strict diet or an intense exercise regime. Yet, the true art lies in the creation of habits that can be sustained beyond the initial enthusiasm; habits that don't feel like an exhaustive effort but like a natural stream carving its way through the bedrock of our daily existence.

We must not ignore the role of our environment in shaping our habits. The availability of nourishing foods, the convenience of exercise options, and the support system within our social and familial circles can all feed into the sustainable practices we wish to cultivate. It is within our power to mold our environment to our benefit.

Let not the anticipation of the journey's length daunt you—the castle was not built in a day, and neither is the fortress of our well-being. Be mindful of the increments, celebrate the small victories; each one is a brick added to the foundation. These triumphs, when strung together, form the robust chain of sustainable habits.

In times of stress or emotional tumult, it is easy to revert to comfort foods and mindless munching. Here, the practice of mindfulness must be our shield and our guide. Recognize the signs, the triggers that may disrupt your well-crafted routine, and have a strategy in place. Perhaps a walk, a conversation with a trusted friend, or a few moments of deep breathing could suffice to steer you away from old haunts.

The nourishment of our bodies, the fuel of our everyday lives, is meant to be a source of joy, not consternation. In the creation of sustainable habits, we seek to find that balance where nutrition meets pleasure, where every meal becomes an opportunity to honor the body and the soul.

Remember, change is an ever-constant companion on the road to wellness. Our habits are not set in stone but are rather the clay that we continuously shape and reshape. Maintaining the plasticity to change them in accord with our growth ensures they will always fit the contours of our evolving lifestyle.

As we draw our musings on sustainable habits to a close, we hope to leave you with a notion of continuity and optimism. To embark upon the journey of mindful eating is to embrace the responsibility we hold for our own well-being—a duty that is both noble and empowering. Set forth with a heart full of courage and an openness to adapt, and you shall find the way to long-lasting success in your health and wellness endeavors.

Chapter 3:
Defining Your Wellness Vision

On the heels of exploring our intricate relationship with food and how our psyche envelopes every bite, we pivot to crystalize a vision that is as individual as our reflection in the still morning lake. Imagine you're standing before a canvas, the colors of nutrition, movement, and mental serenity on your palette, ready to paint your ideal state of wellbeing. It's not mere visualization, but a blueprint of your thriving future laid out with intention and personalized flourish. This vision shouldn't be a far-off dream, nor should it be shrouded in the fog of vagueness. Instead, it's a beacon, encompassing all the radiant colors of your life's spectrum, guiding you through the ebbs and flows of your journey—a lighthouse amidst the tempest of diet myths and fitness fads. A fitness mantra alone can't sculpt it, nor can a singular approach to meal planning truly capture its breadth. It's an elegy and an anthem, a silent promise between you and your potential that whispers of balance, endurance, and the grace of self-acceptance. So, as we embark on this chapter, let's unearth the tools necessary to craft a wellness vision that resonates with your deepest aspirations and catapults you toward a path sprinkled with triumphs and abundant vitality.

Setting Intentions: Goals with Soul

As we wade deeper into the whirling pool of wellness, it becomes evident that robust health is born not only from the corporeal—the nutrients we ingest or the exertion of our muscles—but emerges, quite vibrantly, from the cultivation of our deepest intentions. Thrusting past the superficial allure of numbered goals, this chapter seeks to unearth the rich soil in which Goals with Soul are planted—a realm where resolutions are not merely whispered into existence but are declared with a fiery ardor, their roots entangled with our innermost yearnings.

To set an intention is to kindle a spark within—a prelude to any tangible achievements. It is to converse with our future selves, envisaging a horizon where our well-being burgeons beyond the benchmarks of mere weight loss, fitness, or mental tranquility. This transcendent approach to goal setting avoids the pressure of quantifiable targets and instead encompasses the wholeness of our beings, embedding our aspirations within the fabric of who we are, and more importantly, who we wish to become.

Goals with Soul bear the imprint of authenticity. These are the pulsating dreams that align with your values, that resonate with the very core of your essence. They're not plucked from the latest trends or borrowed from another's journey; rather, they're born from the unique symphony of your life's experiences, desires, and personal revelations. It's less about losing ten pounds or mastering a fitness regime, and more about how you desire to feel in the sunrise of each day—energized, serene, emboldened?

Embarking on this quest necessitates a gentle excavation of self—a reflective pause to consider what wellness truly means to you. Does it whisper of vitality? Does it speak of balance? Or perhaps it sings of resilience. Herein lies the subtlety of this pursuit: that each person's rendition of wellness, like an artful masterpiece, bears distinctive strokes of meaning and substance.

Consider, for a moment, the essence of your motivation. What embers of passion lie dormant, awaiting the revitalizing breath of your attention? Perhaps it's the vigor to play with your children without faltering breath, or the fortitude to scale a mountain, feeling every muscle rejoice in its strength. It could be the serenity of mind that eludes the chaos of modernity, found in silent meditative communion with oneself. This vision, glistening with vitality, is your beacon.

To delineate such goals is a task both wondrous and profound. This soulful approach to intention setting involves a trinity of facets: Clarity, Authenticity, and Emotional Resonance. Clarity demands that you paint your aspirations not with the vagueness of impressionism but with the meticulous detail of a realist. Authenticity requires that your goals are irrevocably bound with your true nature, not a facsimile shaped by societal pressures. Emotional Resonance ensures that your goals pulse with the heartbeat of your most passionate desires, rather than the hollow echo of indifference.

It is pivotal to engrave these intentions into the fiber of your routine. An intention without devoted action is akin to a seed unfavored by sunlight—stunted, unfulfilled. Thus, weave your intentions through the tapestry of your daily life with subtle integrations: a mantra that greets you with the dawn, the embodiment of strength in each mindful meal, the resilience borne of each night's tranquil repose.

The journey towards soulful goals is not one devoid of setbacks or shadowed valleys. Yet, the fortitude we garner from an intention that resonates through our marrow is a lantern illuminating even the most obscure paths. It abides within us, a staunch ally against the tempest of doubt and the quaking ground of unforeseen challenges.

Goals with Soul transform the very ethos of our pursuit. Weight loss transforms from a harsh regimentation to an act of love for one's vessel, fitness metamorphoses into a joyful celebration of capacity, and mental health emerges as the art of nurturing one's inner sanctuary.

This approach beckons a life imprinted with intentional wellness, sparing us the cold embrace of rigid metrics.

As you sculpt your intentions, let them be unfettered by fear or narrow vision. Dream with audacity, for it's in the boundless arenas of our imaginations that the seeds of change are sown. Engage in dialogues with your deepest self, and when your intentions echo back, resonating with the cadence of truth, you'll know that you've set a goal with undeniable soul.

Yet remember, these soulful goals do not exist in isolation. They're part of an intricate web of wellness, woven into the other chapters of this tome. They lay the philosophical foundation upon which your personal path to wellness is built, ensuring that as you venture into nutrition, exercise, and mental wellbeing, your actions are buoyed by an undercurrent of profound purpose.

As you step forward from this chapter, carry with you the sacred knowledge that to set an intention with soul is to embark upon a pilgrimage within. It is a profound commitment to not only achieving but living a fuller, more vibrant version of wellness—one that resonates not just with the body, but with the spirit as well.

Now, let us venture forth with hearts ablaze, set alight by ambitions that soar beyond the tangible—a resounding call to live, to thrive, with intentions that bespeak the language of the soul.

And so, as we weave our narrative through the successive chapters, always bear in mind that the groundwork of soulful intentions precedes the cultivation of sustainable habits, the understanding of one's metabolism, and the embracing of mindfulness in movement. These fierce, burning intents will guide your course with a steady hand, ensuring that you navigate this odyssey with an indomitable spirit and unequivocal grace.

Personalizing Your Path: Wellness is Not One-Size-Fits-All

As we coast gently along the winding path that is your wellness journey, let us pause for a moment to consider an essential truth: the shoes you wear on this trek must fit you, and you alone. Be mindful that your feet are different from those of the fellow beside you or the lady two steps ahead. In matters of health and wellness, you are the craftsman of your own destiny, and indeed, personalization is paramount. This is not only a journey of the body but of the mind and spirit as well.

Consider the sojourners who've traveled this path before you, each with their own set of maps and instruments. Some may have been drawn to the robust exertion of weightlifting, finding solace in the clank of metal and the satisfying exhaustion that follows. Others may have found their solace in the quietude of a yoga studio, breathing in the collective stillness as they stretch towards the sun. Now, it's time for you to find what stirs your soul.

The art of fine-tuning your wellness vision is akin to composing a symphony. Just as a maestro selects each note to create harmony, so must you choose the elements of your wellness routine with intention. Will you begin the day with a burst of energy provided by a morning run, or do you cherish the extra moments in bed, allowing slumber to complete its healing work? Wellness is not prescriptive; rather, it is a manuscript awaiting your personal touch.

As you sculpt your regime, pay heed to the whispers of your body. It speaks a subtle language, nuanced and oft ignored in the hustle of our daily round. Your body speaks of the foods that nourish and those that lead to sluggishness; it reminisces on the joys of movement and the need for rest. To some, a hearty salad brings vibrancy; to others, protein may be the key. Learn the dialect of your own flesh and bone, for in this conversation lies the secret to your wellness.

Survey your past with a detective's eye, charting the moments where wellness eluded you and where it held you in its warm embrace.

These records are not indictments but guiding stars, illuminating the adjustments needed for a bespoke path forward. Have certain diets left you listless, or certain exercises sparked joy? These are the clues that will help you tailor a plan that is yours and yours alone.

In this tapestry of life, your threads may be of varied hues. For some, the rowdy camaraderie of a group fitness class embroiders the edges of their well-being; for others, the solitary challenge of a cold morning swim is what brightens the palette. Rejoice in this diversity and fear not the road less trodden—embrace it.

In the kingdom of wellness, patience reigns supreme. Just as no worthy edifice was built in haste, nor should your vision of health be rushed. Experimentation is the lifeblood of discovery, and it may take a series of trials and errors before your perfect balance is struck. Change one variable at a time—whether it's diet, exercise frequency, or sleep duration—and observe the result with a scientist's curiosity.

Your inner world, too, demands its own unique nourishment. The mind needs silence or perhaps the solace of poignant music; the spirit longs for connection with nature or the kinetic energy of the urban mosaic. Mental and emotional wellness are integral threads in the fabric of your overall well-being, and they too require your attentive care.

There exist industries thriving on the "answer," claiming a monopoly on wellness with rigid regimens and strict diets. But these monoliths overlook the individuality that beats in each of our chests. You must instead become a connoisseur of your own health, sampling and savoring, discarding and embracing, until you find your flavor of vitality.

In the forging of this personal wellness vision, resources abound, promising guidance and support. Yet let not the abundance of navigators dismay you. Instead, sift through these potential allies as you would sift flour for the finest cake, seeking those who will assist in crafting a journey that resonates with the depth of your being.

Just as in life, there will be roadblocks and detours on this wellness odyssey. A cold might derail your fitness routine or a holiday season could tempt you away from balanced eating. Remember, these are but temporary diversions, and your personalized path takes these into account, allowing for flexibility and grace.

In the sacred dance of life, wherein wellness waltzes with our daily demands, setting boundaries is a supreme act of self-love. Your vision may require saying no to late-night work emails to preserve your sleep or eschewing certain social gatherings to ensure your morning meditation remains sacrosanct. Assert these boundaries kindly but firmly, for in them lies the preservation of your health.

As you continue to navigate this chapter in your wellness story, be not swayed by the ephemeral winds of fads or the whisperings of what "everyone else" is doing. The trends will flicker and fade, but your vision, born from the quiet truth of your own experiences, will hold fast. Grounded in authenticity, your path is one that can sustain you through storms and sunshine alike.

In this personalization, there is a profound liberation. No longer caged by ideals that fit as poorly as a borrowed suit, you are free to craft a vision as unique as your fingerprint. Allow your creativity to bloom as you mix and match, continuously shaping a path that brings balance to your body, tranquility to your mind, and joy to your soul.

Let us then embark upon this chapter, not with trepidation but with a joyous heart. Know that in a world rich with variety, your wellness story is yours to write. May it be a tale of discovery, of trials embraced and triumphs savored, a narrative where the wellspring of health bubbles forth in all its splendor—deeply personal, gloriously unique, and entirely yours.

Chapter 4:
Overcoming Weight Loss Plateaus

Just when the symphony of wellness seems to be playing in glorious harmony, weight loss plateaus crash in, uninvited, disrupting the melody we've worked so hard to create. In this transformative Chapter 4, let us dive into the art and science of transcending these baffling stagnations. We've fueled our bodies with mindful nutrition and kindled our spirits with exercise—they're already reveling in the transformation. But the body can be a cunning adversary, sometimes halting progress in its quest for equilibrium. It's natural to feel a twinge of frustration, but this plateau isn't a foe; it's a sign—that our bodies are seeking balance, that they're adapting to our new lifestyles. We'll explore how the deft recalibration of our routines, coupled with the wisdom to acknowledge and embrace the biological handbrake, can fire up the engines of progress once more. From deciphering the quiet language of our metabolisms to deftly tweaking our daily practices, this chapter is your compass to navigate through the doldrums of the plateau and sail into the open waters of continuous personal growth and wellness.

Biological Factors: When Your Body Resists

The journey of weight loss is often painted as a smooth, downhill road, when in reality, it resembles an intricate dance—one step forward, two steps back. Encountering a weight loss plateau is as common as rain in spring, yet it frustrates many an ardent health-seeker. In this faithful confidant that is your quest towards wellness, let's unfold the enigma of your physiology when your body appears to resist the very changes you've been diligently working towards.

Many will whisper to you soft words of simple caloric calculations—burn more than you consume and weight loss is inevitable. But what if the flame seems to wither despite all efforts? That, my friends, is when we must engage in a deeper dialogue with our own biology, an intimate conversation where we acknowledge that weight loss is not merely a matter of willpower. It is a complex interplay between hormones, metabolism, and even genetics.

One such key player in this biological ballad is leptin, a hormone that regulates hunger and satiety. When fat cells shrink, they release less leptin, which the brain may interpret as a starvation signal, thus reducing the metabolic rate and increasing appetite. This is your body's way of preserving itself, akin to a fortress under siege, rationing its resources meticulously.

Metabolic adaptation is another turn in this tale. As you shed pounds, your body requires fewer calories to operate. It becomes more efficient, much like an upgraded machine needing less fuel for the same journey. While commendable in its resourcefulness, this can be an adversary in your battle against the bulge.

The stage of life in which one embarks on a weight loss endeavor also weaves its thread into the narrative. Age-related changes in metabolism notably slow down calorie burning; after all, time leaves none untouched. Additionally, the shifting sands of hormones, for both women and men, cannot be overlooked as they bring about tides of challenge in maintaining or losing weight.

The secret symphony of the gut microbiome also plays its notes in the background. These microscopic maestros can influence how we process food, how we store fat, and even how we crave certain nutrients. The diversity and abundance of this bacterial community are as essential to weight management as the food choices themselves.

Let's not forget the genetic blueprint that each of us carries, the inherited tendencies that can predispose one to a more robust figure or a slender frame. Your genes can influence how your body processes sugars and fats, as well as your propensity for gaining weight in certain areas. Although they are not destiny, they are certainly a voice in the choir of weight management.

Muscle mass is a faithful ally in burning calories even while at rest, yet as weight diminishes, so may muscle, thus reducing the rate at which the body burns energy. Strength training can be a potent countermeasure, encouraging muscle maintenance or growth as you waltz through your weight loss journey.

Hormonal fluctuations that accompany life events such as pregnancy, menopause, or stress can cause your weight loss waltz to feel more like a tango of unpredictability. These periods of life may necessitate a reassessment of strategies and patience as the body recalibrates.

Another often-overlooked factor is sleep quality. Rebuking rest can lead to hormonal imbalances, notably increased ghrelin (the hunger hormone) and decreased leptin (the satiety hormone), leading one to a ravenous state where no calorie seems safe from the onslaught of insatiable hunger.

Underlying medical conditions such as hypothyroidism, polycystic ovary syndrome (PCOS), and insulin resistance are saboteurs stealthily lurking in the shadows, potentially undermining weight loss efforts. Awareness and management of such conditions, often with medical guidance, are crucial to realigning your wellness trajectory.

Regarding medications, certain prescriptions can contribute to weight gain or hinder loss. Everything from antidepressants to beta-blockers has the potential to tip the scales, making vigilant communication with healthcare providers imperative.

Considering these biological factors is to become a master of one's own fate—not to submit to them but to strategize with them in mind. Monitoring not just calorie intake but also nutrient density, maintaining an exercise regime that fosters muscle preservation, attending to one's mental health, and engaging in restorative sleep—these are the rubrics for the enlightened weight-loss journeyman.

Take heart; a plateau does not signify failure. It might simply mean your current lifestyle has become the new equilibrium for your body. This is a sign to reassess, revamp, and reintroduce your body to a novel stimulus—be it dietary, fitness, or lifestyle-oriented—to coax your system into the next chapter of transformation.

Patience must be your ever-present companion, and resilience your armor. Weight loss is not a mere conquest but an ongoing cultivation of the self. Your body is not an adversary but an intricate landscape through which you voyage towards the peak of health and wellness. Sometimes the path goes unseen, but understanding the biological factors at play is akin to wielding a compass; it provides direction when the path ahead is cloaked in the mist of challenge. Onward and upward, the journey continues, with knowledge as your guide and determination as your steed.

Tweaking Your Approach: Strategies to Revitalize Progress

As we navigate the tumultuous tide of weight loss, we often find ourselves at a crossroads, teetering between steadfast resolve and an unnerving plateau. It's in these quiet moments of reflection that the weary traveler of wellness might consider a slight change in direction — a moment to tweak one's approach. Casting aside dismay, let's explore fresh strategies to revitalize progress and recalibrate the compass of health.

First, consider the rhythm of your eating pattern. If the cadence of your meals could speak, would it echo the consistency of a metronome or the erratic beats of a jazz solo? Think about introducing intermittent fasting into your lifestyle, rhythmically oscillating between periods of sustenance and brief sojourns into fasting. Such fluctuations can often shake the doldrums from a stubborn metabolism and ignite a spark within a complacent digestive ballet.

Are you a nocturnal grazer, partaking in a midnight feast as though the moon itself whispered tempting suggestions? Then, my friend, experiment with the kitchen curfew. By closing the pantry's doors as the sun takes its bow, you embark on a nightly fast that extends until the break of dawn. Many have found that this tactic alone plays a harmonious tune on the scales of progress.

Of course, there's the matter of what finds its way onto your plate. If the color palette before you boasts myriad hues akin to a garden in bloom, bravo! Yet, if it's as monochromatic as a winter's day, then enliven your plate with the spectrum found in vegetables and fruits. The profundity of their nutrients dances a merry jig with your bodily functions, optimizing your weight loss opera.

Turn your gaze now upon the potion of life — water. This crystalline nectar is oft overlooked, but its power in breaking a plateau is undeniable. It cleanses, it refreshes, and most importantly, it can aid in staving off an untimely hunger masquerading as thirst. Heighten your fluid intake and watch as it weaves its hydrating spell, flushing away the remnants of stagnation.

If exercise has become as habitual and thoughtless as the brushing of one's teeth, it may be time to ignite a new flame within your regimen. Introduce the vivacity of high-intensity interval training or the stoic art of weightlifting to challenge your physique's status quo. Surprises are not solely for birthdays; your muscles delight in them too.

Do not let sleep be the unsung hero of your journey. If a restful eight-hour slumber is not a part of your nightly soiree, then it's time to RSVP 'yes' to this natural restorative. Sleep weaves its magic most potently when regular and undisturbed, much like the gentle, unfaltering strokes of a painter's brush across the canvas of night.

And what of the pace at which you eat? To dine as if a storm is on your heels edges you closer to overlooking the symphony of flavors. Slow down. Savor each bite as a connoisseur would a fine wine. Mindfulness at the table begets not only pleasure but a deeper connection with satiety's subtle cues.

If your weight loss narrative seems to have become bereft of intrigue, then reintroduce the element of recording. Keep a detailed journal of your daily saga — what you eat, when you eat, and the myriad emotions that swirl around like leaves on an autumn wind. Such chronicling can unveil patterns previously shrouded in the mystery of routine.

And, in a delightful twist, consider the power of spicy foods. As though derived from the mischievous heart of a capsaicin fairy, they spark an internal blaze that can slightly, yet remarkably, burn hotter in the fires of metabolism. An added dash of spice is not merely a treat for the pallet; it's a tactical ally against the common plateau.

Perhaps, then, your palate yearns for the unknown. When was the last time a novel ingredient passed your lips? Diversity in food not only pleases the taste buds but also introduces a party of novel nutrients to your system. New macros and micros can help break through weight loss walls with the gentle but firm determination of roots through soil.

Now, should you find yourself circling the same track, it might be that your body's adaptation is more of a marvel than you realized. It's adept at finding efficiency in repetition. Thus, it's time you penned a new chapter in your workout chronicle. Whether that be through variable resistance training, novel aerobic challenges, or even the grace of a dance class, let each session be a story untold, a mystery unfurled.

Glance, if you will, at the ticking of the clock and align it with your nibbles and noshes. Set meal timing, not just for structure but for synchrony with your circadian rhythms, and discover how the body's intrinsic clock appreciates timely dining.

In the quest for the expulsion of unwanted pounds, it's often a fight not against the grandeur of a banquet but against the minutiae. Tiny bites here, a nibble there, hardly noticed, but cumulatively as weighty as a feast. Take a moment to acknowledge these little transgressions, address them, and behold as the plateau crumbles beneath the newfound integrity of your calorie count.

Finally, provide a mirror to your inner dialogue. What whispers do you entertain that may snuff out the bonfire of ambition? The importance of fostering a positively encouraging mantra cannot be overstressed. Language molds perception, and perception, in turn, forges the reality of your journey. Speak to yourself with kindness, yet with the determination that calls forth action.

With these strategies unfurled like a map across a traveler's table, approach each day as a unique possibility for creation. A gentle tweak here, an experimental twist there, and soon the plateau, once a daunting peak, becomes a distant memory, a mere pitstop in the grand voyage of health and wellness. So, gently encourage these changes upon the stage of your routine and watch with patient excitement as the weight loss narrative once again surges with life and vigorous momentum.

Chapter 5:
Stress Management for Sustainable Weight Loss

Like an insidious whisper that undermines the harmony of our wellness efforts, stress stands as an invisible antagonist in the narrative of our health. Stress doesn't merely ripple through our mental poise; it plunges into our physical reservoirs, often tipping the scales away from the coveted equilibrium where weight loss thrives. Yet, within our grasp lies the arsenal to parry its thrusts. The dance of stress hormones—those covert saboteurs of our metabolism—can be artfully managed, steering our bodily systems back to a place where weight loss isn't a battle but a natural consequence of our newfound serenity. Enlist meditation's gentle power to quiet the tempestuous seas of the mind, and embrace deep breathing's rhythmic lull to anchor your presence in the here and now. With each intentional breath, we teach our body the language of peace, potentially transforming the arduous journey of shedding pounds into a walk in the park—a park bathed in warm light and the tranquility of attainable, enduring weight loss.

The Stress-Weight Nexus: Making the Connection

As the pages of our wellness narrative turn, we find ourselves at a compelling chapter, an intersection of tolls – the remarkable relationship between stress and weight. It is a tapestry of influence where one's mental storms can cast shadows over the physical self, often in the form of unwelcome weight. Indeed, the stress-weight nexus is not a myth concocted by worried minds, but a tangible connection that science has traced with earnest precision.

Consider stress as the invisible puppeteer, one that can control appetite and metabolism with such finesse that you may not even realize the strings attached. The mechanisms of this control are biochemical in nature, involving a hormonal cast comprising primarily of cortisol, the notorious stress hormone. When stress elevates, so too does cortisol, and it's here that the plot thickens. Elevated cortisol can signal the body to store fat, particularly around the abdomen, and simultaneously whisper sweet urges to seek comfort in foods – typically those rich in fats and sugars.

Yet, it's not just about the direct hormonal effects; stress also weaves its way into behaviors. It's the hurried meals snatched between commitments, the emotional eating when the world's weight feels on your shoulders, or the cravings that echo during late-night musings – all are threads in the stress-weight tapestry. In a way, stress can disrupt the natural ebb and flow of appetite regulation, pushing you towards a cycle of overeating and weight gain that feels maddeningly difficult to escape.

Moreover, let's not overlook sleep – that restorative sanctuary. Stress can be a thief in the night, stealing sleep and with it, the body's opportunity to balance and repair. Poor sleep doesn't just lead to fatigue; it's a partner in crime with stress, resulting in a further hormonal upheaval that can sabotage weight management. The cortisol predicament is agitated further by imbalances in leptin and ghrelin, hormones that tell you when to eat and when to stop. Add sleep deprivation to the mix, and you've primed the body for weight gain.

But there's another side to this nexus to contemplate – the role of chronic stress. While acute stress can lead to temporary weight fluctuations, it's the enduring, perpetual stress that builds an abode in your daily life that truly entrenches the weight issue. Chronic stress can perpetuate high cortisol levels, impacting not only appetite and cravings but also your very metabolism, leading to what feels like a slowed grind, hindering weight loss efforts significantly.

It's essential to recognize that everyone's stress response is as unique as their fingerprint. What sends one person into a cortisol surge might barely register to another. This variance is born of genetic makeup, environmental factors, and past experiences. And so, your personal stressors demand a tailor-made approach to untie the knots that lead to weight gain.

At this juncture, you might feel the weight of this information, but let's pivot towards empowerment. Understanding the stress-weight nexus is your first step in disarming it. Awareness can light the path to strategies such as mindfulness techniques and stress management, which we'll delve into further in this journey of wellness.

Think of stress as a call to action; now that you know its impact on weight, you're equipped to take that call. Stress management isn't just about reducing the mental load. It's about altering physiological responses, breaking the cycle of stress eating, and renegotiating the terms with your metabolism.

Embrace this knowledge with the appreciation that managing stress is not merely beneficial for your mental health but is a cornerstone of sustainable weight management. Readdressing the balance of your life's scales – the physical and the psychological – can shift your weight narrative towards a tale of triumph.

Let's also not underestimate the environment's role in the nexus. It is the stage upon which stress and weight interact, where external pressures, societal expectations, and personal demands commingle to influence the outcome. In controlling your environment – such as basic organization and time management – you reclaim some measure of control over the stress that flows into your life.

Education is an ally in this battle. With knowledge comes the power to make informed decisions – about what you eat, how you respond to stress, and how you can implement changes. This clarity can be the guiding light towards healthier choices rather than succumbing to the impulse-borne decisions shaped by stress.

It's also about redefining the concept of comfort. The comfort foods that stress lures us toward offer but a fleeting solace. The true comfort is found in the equilibrium of a balanced life, where mind and body align in harmony. Identifying more constructive avenues to comfort yourself – such as physical activity, social interaction, and hobbies – creates a buffer against the siren call of stress eating.

Ultimately, making the connection between stress and weight is a call to holistic action. It is about harmonizing the internal with the external, understanding that the weight one carries is not just of the body, but also of the mind. As we delve deeper into mindfulness techniques and strategies for stress relief, you will find that managing stress encompasses both the silencing of mental cacophony and the tuning of the body's rhythms.

So, while stress may tip the scales, know that equanimity and mindfulness can balance them once more. Weaving together threads of knowledge, behavior change, and stress management creates a tapestry resilient enough to withstand the pressures that once led to weight gain. The stress-weight nexus, once demystified, becomes not a foe, but a landscape of understanding where sustainable weight loss can flourish.

Thus, in managing stress, you do not simply chase away the specter that haunts your scales. You invite a profound transformation that resonates through every facet of your being – strengthening, fortifying, and ultimately, liberating. Stand firm in this connection, and watch as the scales tip in favor of a wellness that transcends the physical, becoming an emblem of a life richly lived and mindfully balanced.

Mindfulness Techniques: Breathing, Meditation, and Beyond

Navigating the turbulent seas of weight management, one might understand the profound influence of stress—its swells and dips can wash over our best intentions, topple our discipline, and leave us floundering in the wake of emotional eating and hormonal turbulence. Taming this tempest is essential, and mindfulness is our most stalwart ally in this quest. It's an anchor, allowing us to pause, to breathe, to observe—and importantly, to choose.

The act of breathing, seemingly so mundane, is the cornerstone of mindfulness. Envision the breath as a brushstroke on the canvas of consciousness, each inhale a swath of light, every exhale a release of shadow. The discipline of *focused breathing* is simple in concept but profound in impact. By merely attending to the rhythm of one's breath, by feeling the rise and fall of the chest or the belly, by hearing the whisper of air in and out, one can anchor oneself in the now. Amidst stress, this focus can be a lifeline back to equilibrium.

Meditation, a word that intimates serenity to some and vexes others with its promise of stillness, is a crucial flourish in our strategy for stress management. Meditation is not the art of silencing the mind—as anyone who has attempted it can attest—but rather the practice of observing without attachment. In the cathedral of our thoughts, meditation teaches us to sit on the pews and watch the procession of feelings and sensations without joining the parade.

There are myriad forms of meditation, from the measured cadences of *Transcendental Meditation* to the mindful awareness of *Zen*. For weight management, techniques such as *Mindful Eating Meditation* heighten our awareness of hunger cues and taste satisfaction, serving as a bulwark against the autopilot of overeating.

Progressing beyond breath and mental discipline, mindful practices can encompass all manner of experiences. Consider the art of *yoga*, a dance between movement and stillness, each pose a testament to the moment's fleeting nature. With each stretch and hold, the yogi becomes more intimately acquainted with the nuances of their physical form and the present's quiet voice.

Even for those skeptical of yoga's charms, the broader church of mindfulness offers other pursuits. The simple practice of walking in nature, when done with presence, can serve as a salve for a stressed spirit and a body aching from the sedentary shackles of modern life.

Rituals, too, have their place in this tapestry of techniques. A morning routine infused with mindfulness—a few minutes spent savoring the warmth of a shower, the ritual of preparing a nutritious breakfast, or simply sitting with a cup of tea before the day begins—can fortify the mind against stress's storm.

The alchemy of mindfulness is its ability to transmute the mundane into the meaningful. Chores and daily tasks become opportunities for practice. The act of washing dishes, folding laundry, or even waiting in line can become a moment for mindfulness, turning a potentially frustrating wait into an opportunity to check in with one's body and mind.

Journaling, often overlooked, is an exercise in mindfulness for those who find solace in words. Pouring one's thoughts onto paper provides distance to observe one's internal landscape—a practice that can illuminate patterns and stressors contributing to weight gain.

While the tapestry of mindfulness and its diverse threads offers solace and strength, it is also a skill—a muscle that requires consistent flexing. The integration of mindfulness into one's life isn't a one-time act but a cultivation of habit. It's a garden that needs regular tending to flourish.

Consider also the power of *guided imagery*, a technique of meditation where one visualizes a serene environment or a desired outcome. For those embroiled in the challenge of weight loss, envisioning oneself as healthier and at peace can be a potent motivator and a means to reinforce one's commitment to wellness.

It's important to acknowledge that the journey through mindfulness is a personal one, and what serves as a sanctuary for one person may not resonate with another. It's about finding the methods that speak to one's soul and fit within the cadence of one's daily life. The key is to explore these techniques with an open mind and patience.

When applied to the sphere of sustainable weight loss, mindfulness transforms the experience from one of deprivation and struggle to one of awareness and growth. Stress, that cunning villain which so often derails our weight management efforts, can be moderated and its impacts lessened through these practices.

Emerging scientific literature affirms what many practitioners have experienced first-hand: that mindfulness can recalibrate our relationship with food, improve dietary choices, and facilitate a more harmonious interaction with our own bodies. It's about molding our internal dialogue from one of criticism and denial to one of acceptance and nourishment.

Ultimately, it is critical not to underestimate the ripple effects of such techniques. The implementation of mindfulness in stress management is not merely about achieving a specific weight goal; it's about nurturing a lasting state of mental well-being that echoes into every aspect of our wellness journey. It is a path to empower hearts and minds, as much as it shapes bodies.

Know that embarking on the path of mindfulness is not an instantaneous remedy. It is a gradual process, a learning curve that bends toward a horizon of enlightened self-care and thoughtful weight management. It's a journey best embarked upon with the understanding that each day brings new challenges, and with it, new opportunities to practice the art of presence.

Chapter 6:
The Exercise-Mindfulness Connection

In the preceding chapters, we've woven a tapestry of vitality, with mindfulness as the recurring thread enhancing each wellness aspect. In Chapter 6, we delve into the intricate symbiosis between exercise and mindfulness, a liaison as vital to the mind as it is to sinew and bone. This partnership fosters an acute awareness of our physical form and the rhythm of our thoughts amidst the ebb and flow of movement. Imagine the experience of exercise transformed—a run not merely a pounding of pavement but a harmonious dance between breath and stride; strength training not solely a series of repetitions but an exploration of the body's silent language. Through this chapter, we open the door to mindful movement, exploring how each squat, stretch, or step can be imbued with intention and presence. This isn't just sweat and burn; it's a dialogue with the self, a merging of corporeal effort and mental clarity that can heighten the efficacy of your wellness regimen. As you embark on your fitness ventures, remember, it's the unity of body and mind that propels you toward peak health and unwavering mental fortitude.

Mindful Movement: Exercise as a Meditative Practice

Embarking on the journey of wellness, where every stride and breath intertwine harmoniously, we arrive at a crossroads of body and mind.

Picture, if you will, a form of physical articulation so serene it becomes akin to meditation, transforming exercise from a mere task to an enveloping experiential practice: this is the essence of mindful movement.

To walk this path, you needn't summon the strength of Hercules, nor the serenity of a Tibetan monk. What's required is just a vigilant presence and conscious engagement with each muscular contraction and extension. Engaged in such a manner, you'll find that the monotony of exercise dissipates, much like morning mist under the gentle touch of the sun's rays.

If you've ever lost yourself in the rhythmical motion of walking or felt the ebb and flow of your breath while swimming, you've tasted the sweet bliss of mindful movement. Such practices encapsulate not only the physical choreography but also weave in the subtle threads of intention, focus, and acute awareness.

The pulsing heartbeat during a jog can morph into a drummer's cadence, guiding you into a deeper state of consciousness. It's in the synchronization of your body's movements and your breath's rhythm that you uncover a state of heightened awareness, often elusive in our quotidian bustle.

Consider the intricate dance of tai chi, a martial art that epitomizes the grace of mindful movement, where every gesture is deliberate and soaked in attentiveness. While the outer world whirls in its perpetual carousel, the practitioner remains centered, witnessing each turn of the wrist, each subtle shift of weight.

Similarly, the practice of yoga unfurls as a tapestry of mindful movement. As one transitions from posture to posture—a sequence of physical poetry—one must marry movement to breath. And in the silent spaces between inhales and exhales, one discovers the stillness that is as vast and deep as the night sky.

What of resistance training—the clinking of weights and the rhythm of repetitions? Even here, amidst the sinewy symphony of effort, there exists an opportunity for mindfulness. By tuning into the sensation of muscle fibers contracting, by feeling the weight in your hands as something more than steel and rubber, we transform the repetitious into the revelatory.

Do not think that to engage in this practice you must scale the peaks of extreme exertion. Mindful movement is not confined to vigorous activity. Even in the gentlest stroll or the most unassuming stretch, there is room for presence. To be mindful is to dwell fully in the moment of movement, no matter the intensity.

In our daily rush, we often succumb to the temptation of 'getting it over with,' reducing exercise to a checkmark on our ever-growing list of to-dos. Mindful movement implores you to shun such haste. It calls you to experience each motion in its entirety, to savor the journey as much as the destination.

Indeed, cultivating mindfulness in motion can serve as an anchor in the turbulent seas of daily life. Just as the ebb and flow of the ocean's waves are a testament to nature's rhythm, so too can our own rhythmic movements ground us in the present.

Such a practice is not merely for the lithe and limber. Mindful movement extends its hand to all, irrespective of age, flexibility, or strength. It asks only for your attention and willingness to journey inward, exploring the space within each breath, each step, each stretch.

Is it not wondrous then, that through the depths of physical engagement we can access the innermost corridors of our psyche? By entwining the threads of mindfulness with the sinews of our being, we weave together a tapestry of inner harmony and external vitality.

Learn to listen—to the whispered cues of your body, to the silent anthem of your breath. This is the hallowed conversation between you and the corpus that carries you. Through this dialogue, through the recognition and appreciation of the body's language, you reclaim a sense of sovereignty over your own being.

To embark on this odyssey of mindful movement is to step into a realm where fitness transcends the physical and becomes a conduit for mental clarity and emotional equilibrium. It is a journey of self-discovery, a crusade without conquest, where the spoils are inner tranquility and a profound connection with the vessel that is your body.

As we continue to unravel the intricacies of the exercise-mindfulness connection in subsequent chapters, remember to integrate the principles of mindful movement. Embrace your body's capabilities, push gently at the edges of your limitations, and let every movement be a meditation—an affirmation of life and an ode to the splendor of existence.

Finding Your Flow: Incorporating Mindful Fitness

As we traverse the path of harmonizing exercise with inner tranquility, finding your flow with mindful fitness emerges as a beacon of serene potency. Imagine a seamless blend of motion and stillness, where every sinew and synapse aligns in purposeful action. This is not merely about sweating; it's about awakening to the rapture of your true physical potential, harmonized with a calm and present mind.

Embarking on mindful fitness is akin to learning a new dialect of the body's language. It requires attentiveness to the subtle dialogues of muscles and breath, of heartbeat and intention. As you engage in your chosen form of physical exertion, channel your focus inward. Observe the sensations coursing through your limbs, the rhythm of your respiration, the way your feet kiss the earth with every stride.

Envision yoga, for example. Beyond its stretch and pose, it is a dance of breath and movement, a silent symphony that resonates within the hollows of the self. Each asana is an act of mindfulness, a hold that anchors you firmly in the moment. Yet, the true fluidity is found not in the holding, but in the transitions, the grace-filled journey from one posture to another.

Similarly, consider the cadence of a jogger. The solitary percussion of feet padding against the path can metamorphose into a meditative jaunt. With each inhalation and exhalation synced to the rhythm of movement, the jogger's mind clears, allowing for an experience rich with presence and devoid of the day's clutter.

Integrating mindful fitness into your regimen need not be constrained by the walls of a sanctuary of calm such as a yoga studio. Indeed, even the din and clatter of a gym can provide the backdrop for a mindful lifting session. Here, amidst the symphony of clinking weights, you can zero in on the tension and release of every muscle group, the controlled breaths fueling your strength, and the exquisite precision of your form.

When we talk about flow, it's more than a mere state of mind—it's akin to a river cutting through a landscape, effortless yet powerful. Attain this flow by immersing yourself in the task at hand, letting all else fade into the periphery. Whether it's cycling, swimming, or dance, let the activity consume your focus completely, so that you and the movement are indivisible.

The benefits of mindful exercise extend far beyond the physicality. While your body carves out strength and stamina, your mind cultivates resilience and calmness. This confluence of physical and mental fortitude plays a pivotal role in maintaining weight loss, fitness, and overall mental health.

As you delve into mindful fitness, remember to set realistic goals. These goals should be nurtured patiently and without self-judgment. Progress may be incremental, but it's progress nonetheless. Each day on the mat or the track is another stitch in the tapestry of your wellness journey.

To truly incorporate mindfulness into your fitness routine, you'll also want to pay heed to your body's whispers and roars. Observe any discomfort, acknowledging it without fear, and mindfully adapting your movements to accommodate, not aggravate.

Furthermore, don't underestimate the power of visualization. Picture each workout as a narrative where you're both the protagonist and the scribe. Visualize success and let that image guide you through each repetition and set, instilling your efforts with purpose and direction.

It's important, too, to savor the moments after your exercise—what athletes call the 'afterglow.' Bask in the ethereal calm that cloaks your senses, the lovely fatigue that whispers of a job well done. This quiet contemplation is as integral to mindful fitness as the exercise itself.

For those embarking on this path, don't look for a transformation overnight. The evolution of your body and mind is a journey that meanders, with hills and valleys. Patience and persistence are your steadfast companions, shepherding you towards a horizon brimming with health and balance.

Beginners should start slow, weaving mindfulness into their practice in increments. Perhaps it begins with five minutes of focused breathing before a run, or it could be the conscious release of tension during a stretching sequence. Let the practice grow organically from these tender roots.

The interlude between exercises is ripe for mindfulness as well. Seize these moments for mindful reflection. Assess how your body feels, what it's telling you, and how your breath can act as a vehicle for relaxation and recovery.

Ultimately, mindful fitness is a tapestry woven with the threads of your own experiences, beliefs, and goals. It's a symphony with a tempo unique to you. And as you find your flow, let the practice sculpt not just a healthier body, but a sanctuary of peace and strength within you.

May this journey through mindful movement foster not just a transcendent rapport between muscle and mind, but also illuminate the overarching truth: that the pursuit of health is an act of profound self-care, a poetic tending to the garden of one's own well-being.

Chapter 7:
Nutritional Balance for Optimal Health

Transitioning gracefully from the art of mindful fitness to the science of sustenance, we unfold the pivotal chapter of our wellness journey—**Nutritional Balance for Optimal Health**. The very fabric of our being is stitched together with the threads of what we consume; thus, we must weave with intention. It isn't enough to merely fill our plates; we must question, what are we truly nourishing? You see, the macronutrient dance of carbs, proteins, and fats is one of delicate balance—a waltz that requires finesse and understanding to maintain the body's harmony. It's about crafting a colorful tapestry with greens and grains, not merely because we ought, but because our bodies yearn for the lush vibrancy they provide. Let's not embark on this leg of the journey with thoughts of restriction but rather with the zest of adding value to each morsel that passes our lips. For it is in the wholesome plenty that we find the keys to unlock our optimal state—a veritable Eden where weight loss, fitness, and mental health coexist in perfect equilibrium.

Macronutrient Mastery: Carbs, Proteins, and Fats

Continuing from where we paused, let's delve into the pillars of our nutritional castle – carbohydrates, proteins, and fats. Each macro-nutrient holds the key to unlocking a realm of wellness, where health and vitality sit enthroned. Let's first wander through the lush fields of carbohydrates. They are the swift heralds of energy, delivering glucose to our bodily kingdom near and far. Yet, not all carbs are born equal. Imagine the vast difference between the sturdy wholesomeness of ancient grains and the fleeting sweetness of a sugared confection. Whole, unprocessed carbohydrates are akin to a trusty steed, providing sustained energy, while refined sugars are more like a tempestuous charger – quick to bolt, leaving havoc in its wake.

Moving on, proteins enter the stage. They are the robust warriors repairing our tissues and fortifying our defenses. These valiant molecules are found in abundance in both palace and pasture – whether in the form of a knight's leg of lamb or a peasant's pot of beans. Proteins are essential for a multitude of functions, from constructing the very fibers of our muscles to crafting the enzymes that govern every chemical reaction within our borders. Just as every knight has a different crest, proteins come in various forms, with amino acids being the unique heraldry that distinguishes them.

Fats, once shunned like outcasts, have now been welcomed back into the realm, recognized for their splendor and necessity. They are the monarchs of satiety, ruling over our appetite with a benevolent hand. Found in nuts, seeds, fish, and quality oils, fats are essential to cushion our organs, construct our cell membranes, and serve as a reserve of energy in times of scarcity. They come bearing gifts of fat-soluble vitamins and essential fatty acids, which our bodies, like wise rulers, cannot produce on their own.

Yet beware, not all fats reign with wisdom and grace. Trans fats and some saturated fats are the maleficent rulers of the fat kingdom, lurking in processed foods and waiting to besiege our heart's stronghold. It's our duty to choose allies wisely and favor those who govern with our health in mind – the monounsaturated and polyunsaturated fats.

To wield these macronutrients with mastery, we must understand the balance and harmony required for our individual constitutions. A symphony of balanced eating sees the carbohydrates' lilting melody harmonize with the steady rhythm of proteins, all under the resonant bass of healthy fats. When this balance is achieved, the body thrives, and we find our optimal form, fueling our adventures in fitness and mental health.

In habit's fortress, the balance can easily be toppled – too much of noble protein, and the kidneys may protest; an overindulgence in bulky fats, yet the gallant liver might rebel. Carbohydrates, in excess, can cause the village storehouses to overflow, leading to unwanted wastage - or worse, the onset of metabolic dissent. This delicate dance of macronutrients is both an art and a science, requiring mindfulness and intent.

It's easy to become lost in the maze of nutritional advice, where every turn brings a new diet decree or forbidden fruit. But remember, nourishment is a personal journey and what works for one may lead another astray. It's essential to listen to your own body's whispers and roars, serving it with the respect befitting a royal court. Are you listening when it signals satiety or are you by chance drowning out its voice in a sea of plenty?

Consider carbohydrates our primary fuel source. They're the kingdom's bustling commerce, trading for immediate energy and storing for later use. Yet amidst the constant chattering markets, ensure your coins are spent wisely. Invest in complex carbs found in fruits, vegetables, and whole grains, and be wary of the seemingly attractive but often deceptive refined carbs and sugars.

Proteins, on the other hand, are the builders and repairers. They're the blacksmiths and carpenters tending to our body's infrastructure. While the amount of protein required will vary depending on one's station – whether a laborer or a lady of leisure – it's crucial to supply the body with enough material to maintain and repair the ramparts of our health.

Fats, the regal rulers of our nutrient kingdom, must be chosen with discretion. Seek out those who provide long-term prosperity – like omega-3 and omega-6 fatty acids from fish, nuts, and seeds. They are the essential diplomats negotiating processes from inflammation to cognition.

In pursuit of harmonious health, we mustn't be enticed by flamboyant feasting rituals that promise quick victories. These often lead down treacherous paths clouded by poor nutrition and imbalanced diets. True mastery lies in a diverse array of whole foods, providing all the macronutrients a wise ruler and hearty subject might need.

Even as we focus on these macronutrients, we mustn't forget the kingdom's unsung heroes – fiber, vitamins, and minerals. They're the tireless stewards and handmaids ensuring the smooth running of our daily lives. Their story is told elsewhere in this tome, but remember, their roles are interwoven with our stately trio of macros.

To orchestrate such a banquet of nutrients, one must also become a vigilant gatekeeper. Each morsel of food crossing your lips should be considered - does it serve your health, or is it merely a court jester, distracting you with taste while offering little substance?

Let us approach our plates with the wisdom of a seasoned sage, constructing meals that bring honor to our bodies. By achieving macronutrient mastery, we set forth on a path of optimal health, where every fortification is strong, and every citizen within prospers. Our quests for weight loss, fitness, and mental well-being are all championed by this knowledgeable command of carbs, proteins, and fats. Thus armed, we march forward in the quest for lasting wellness – with balance as our banner and vitality as our steed.

The Power of Plants: Integrating More Greens

As we've delved deeply into the intricacies of macronutrients, let us turn our gaze to the bountiful garden of nutrition that awaits our discovery. Vegetation, in its most natural state, offers us a cacophony of benefits that transcend the realm of mere vitamins and minerals. Greens, verdant and robust, are more than just a splash of color on our plates; they are the cornerstone of vitality and balance in our diets.

For centuries, plants have held a revered place in the domain of health, trusted as nature's apothecaries. They harbor within them a symphony of phytonutrients, fibers, and antioxidants, whose roles in our bodily orchestra are as crucial as they are varied. Integrating more greens into our meals is not a mere act of nourishment; it is an embrace of life's essence, a chorus of wellness singing through every cell.

Consider the leafy greens: spinach, kale, and Swiss chard. These are the titans of nutrition, flexing their muscle through high levels of iron, calcium, potassium, and magnesium. But their power extends beyond these elements; they contain compounds that may help protect us against the vagaries of age and disease. Lutein and zeaxanthin, found abundantly within their fibers, stand as vigilant guardians of our sight, helping to fend off the ravages of macular degeneration.

Moreover, greens are integral to the management of one's weight. Low in calories yet rich in fiber, they fill the belly's expanse without tipping the scales, thus promoting satiety and discouragement of overindulgence. They are the gallant knights in the ongoing battle against unwanted pounds, holding the line with poise and determination.

Yet, the question lingers: how might one weave these green threads through the tapestry of their daily diet? The answer lies in creativity. Start your day with a smoothie, vibrant and green, with baby spinach or kale blended into your favorite fruits. This concoction is not only a feast for the senses but also a send-off into the day that is both energizing and aligned with our health goals.

Lunch could be a salad that is anything but pedestrian. Imagine a bed of mixed greens, resplendent with the colors of cherry tomatoes and the crunch of seeds and nuts. Drizzle it with a dressing of olive oil and apple cider vinegar, a combination that whispers of rustic charm and culinary wisdom, and you have a meal that delights while it sustains.

Come dinner, greens need not play a mere supporting role but might take center stage. Let collard greens be wrapped around a melody of quinoa and vegetables, or let the heartiness of cooked mustard greens complement the smoky richness of grilled tempeh. The possibilities are endless, bound only by the imagination and one's adventurous palate.

Do not neglect the world of herbs. Their potency lies not just in their flavors but in their health benefits. Basil, cilantro, parsley, and more, these culinary mainstays are packed with unique properties that may support our immune systems, combat inflammation, and even lift our spirits with their enchanting aromas.

And as we talk of spirits, let us not forget the role of greens in our mental well-being. The vibrant hues and life-affirming qualities of vegetables have been shown to enhance mood and provide a visual reminder of the Earth's abundance. The act of preparing and consuming them can be as much a meditation as any mantra or mindful breath.

We also advocate for sustainability, for greens present us with the perfect opportunity to support local agriculture. Seasonal vegetables procured from local farmers' markets find their way into our bellies, but first, they enrich our lives with their tales of origin, stories entwined with the very soil of our community. Thus, integrating more greens is not merely a dietary choice but a commitment to the planet and its future.

However, let us not be naïve to the barriers that stand in our way. The modern lifestyle is beleaguered by convenience and pre-packaged solutions that often leave greens by the wayside. It takes an act of willful defiance to choose the fresh over the processed, to take the few extra minutes to prepare a vegetable-laden meal when a pre-made dish beckons with its siren call of immediacy.

It is here that we find the true test of our dedication to health. Must we not rise to the challenge, to renew our vows with every crunch of a crisp lettuce leaf, with every sip of a green smoothie? For to integrate greens into our lives is no passive act; it is a declaration, a powerful affirmation of our commitment to the temple that is our body.

Throughout this journey, it is crucial to remember balance. Greens are the stars of this chapter, yet they find their fullest expression when accompanied by a chorus of whole grains, lean proteins, and healthy fats. It is in the harmony of food groups that we discover the symphony of nutrition that can sustain, heal, and energize.

To conclude, let us partake in the power of plants with reverence and joy. May we find in every leaf and every stem, the keys to unlocking optimal health. Integrate greens, and watch as the colors of vitality paint themselves across the canvas of your life, promising a future of wellness illuminated by the natural brilliance of the Earth's gifts.

Chapter 8:
The Support System: Nurturing Wellness Together

Embarking on a quest for wellness is akin to setting sail on a vast, uncharted ocean—the journey is infinitely more manageable with a sturdy vessel and a devoted crew. In this essential chapter, we dive into the profound depths of community and companionship that bolster our resolve and nourish our determination to thrive. Our tribe, the unsung heroes in our narrative of health, provides emotional ballast and wisdom in unsteady times, making each shared triumph and challenge a layered stone in the foundation of our collective well-being. We shall explore, not just the wide tapestry of familial kinship, friends, and confidants that fortify our spirits, but also the invaluable guidance of seasoned professionals who illuminate the path toward our most vibrant selves. In the harmony of shared experiences and the symphony of concerted efforts, there lies an immeasurable strength that empowers each of us to rise above solitary struggles and embrace a future of wellness, crafted together, in unwavering solidarity.

Building Your Tribe: The Strength of Community

Embarking on the road to wellness is akin to setting sail on a vast and sometimes turbulent sea. The journey, while enriching, can promise both swells of triumph and waves of setbacks. Yet, no captain of any ship need navigate the ocean's whims alone. Herein lies the crux of our current meditation: the immeasurable value of building a tribe, a steadfast community that shores up our resolve and buoys our spirits in the pursuit of health and wellness.

The wisdom in pooling our resources is self-evident; as social beings, our evolutionary tapestry is woven with threads of camaraderie and mutual support. A tribe offers more than mere companionship; it provides a network of accountability, a platform to share knowledge, and the collective strength to propel us forward in our wellness endeavors.

Let's ponder the inception of such a tribe. It springs to life from the seeds of commonality, nurtured by shared goals, and fertilized by the will to succeed. It's not just about finding people who are on the same path but about curating a circle that respects, encourages, and challenges one another in equal measure.

We begin by seeking those who resonate with our purpose, who understand the ebbs and flows of our journey. This could be a group dedicated to fitness, a community centered around mindful eating, or a collective committed to stress reduction. Whichever the focus, the unity in diversity allows for a rich tapestry of perspectives, each one providing unique insights into our shared ordeal.

Moreover, in constructing this fellowship, we must not overlook the magic of inclusivity. A tribe that embraces a variety of backgrounds and perspectives is not just richer in culture but robust in its ability to navigate the multifaceted nature of wellness. It's important that within our tribe, voices are not only heard but celebrated, crafting an atmosphere where all members feel valued and empowered.

As we lay the foundation for this community, let us also acknowledge the importance of open dialogue. Communication facilitates the sharing of triumphs and defeats alike, allowing us to feel seen and understood. It's through these exchanges that we foster deeper connections, turning acquaintances into allies in our wellness journey.

But a tribe is more than just a supportive cheering squad; it's also a wellspring of inspiration. Witnessing the strides others make in their wellness ventures can ignite a spark of motivation within us, spur innovation in our own methods, and even bring about unanticipated breakthroughs in how we approach our health.

The process of goal setting within a community also helps in materializing our ambitions. A goal shared is a vision given wings, and within the bounds of a tribe, these aspirations take flight through collaborative effort and mutual encouragement. It's a potent reminder that our individual successes contribute to the elevation of the collective wellbeing.

Collaboration within the tribe yields practical benefits as well. Pooling resources, be it in the form of shared knowledge, exercise equipment, or healthful recipes, enhances the efficiency of our wellness endeavors. This collective repository of tools and experiences becomes an invaluable asset, one that each member can draw upon and contribute to.

It's also vital to remember that part of community strength is acknowledging when a member's load becomes too hefty to shoulder alone. In these moments, the tribe's role shifts from fellow pilgrim to a sanctuary of solace, wherein the burden is lightened by the hands of many, offering relief and respite to the wearied traveler.

There's also an ironclad bond formed through shared vulnerability; as we open up about our struggles with weight loss, fitness, or mental health, we grant permission for our peers to do the same. This exchange of truth forges a trust that holds the framework of the tribe together—a safety net for when we falter and a celebratory banner for when we flourish.

In the cultivation of such community, we find not only solace but also a mirror reflecting our own growth. Each individual's transformation becomes a collective metamorphosis, with every personal breakthrough contributing to the elevation of the tribe as a whole.

Now, let us not be naïve to assume that conflict shan't ever darken our doorstep. Indeed, within any group, discord may arise, and yet, it is through tackling and resolving these differences that the tribe strengthens and matures. In navigating these challenges, we unveil new layers of understanding and practice the very essence of wellness: balance and harmony.

In the delicate dance of give and take, where support waxes and wanes like the phases of the moon, it becomes evident that the role we play within our tribe is not static but ever-evolving. There are times when we are the rock upon which others may lean and times when we are the reed, bending with the winds of our own trials, relying on the steadfastness of our community.

In conclusion, the tapestry of a thriving tribe is interwoven with threads of empathy, trust, inspiration, and unwavering support. As we each continue to tread the ever-winding paths of wellness and self-discovery, let us acknowledge that the strength of our tribe is an integral beacon of light. It guides us through the fog of uncertainty and stands as a monument to the collective power of shared journeys and intertwined destinies in the quest for health.

Professional Guidance: When to Seek Help

The winding road of wellness, with its profound personal victories and its occasional challenging ravines, isn't meant for solitary travelers. Along your journey, you may find that guidance from professionals can illuminate paths that were once shrouded in mist. Knowing when to seek help frames the journey as a shared adventure rather than a lonesome trek.

Embarking on a journey of health and wellness often begins with boundless enthusiasm. Yet at times, you may stumble upon unexpected hurdles. When the scale ceases to budge despite your endeavors, or when the mirror reflects a stranger cloaked in stress and fatigue, the counsel of a healthcare professional isn't merely a luxury; it becomes a necessity.

Imagine yourself nurturing a seedling, tender and full of promise. As it pushes through the earth, you must decide: When is the right time to seek the wisdom of a gardener? The parallels between cultivating your wellness and a thriving plant are striking. While sunlight and water might suffice for a time, there will come days when the soil needs the keen eye of a master to detect deficiencies and prescribe remedies.

When fluctuations in mood shadow over your typical sunshine, or when anxiety thrums through your veins, a mental health professional could offer the lantern to light your way. They stand as lighthouses casting their beams upon oceans stormy with worry and doubt. Acknowledge your feelings, for they are the compass directing you towards those who can help navigate the tempestuous seas of mental stress.

Moreover, if whispers of pain thread their way through your days, winding tightly around your joys and choking them into silence, the expertise of a medical professional is paramount. Pain is the body's clarion call, signaling that it's time to seek assistance that transcends your foundational knowledge. Refusing to heed these calls can lead the discomfort to embed itself deeper, becoming a silent stowaway on your journey.

Within the realm of fitness and weight loss, when progress stalls and the path forward seems muddied by a plateau, a personal trainer or a nutritionist can serve as your compass. They come with maps in hand—regimens and meal plans charted out with precision, ready to steer you back on course towards the horizon of your goals.

If you find your plate perpetually overflowing with tasks, your breaths short, and sleep elusive, it's time to consider the guidance of a stress management counselor. They offer strategies crafted to return you to a harbor of tranquility amid the storm of daily obligations. Clasping their hand is a step towards calmer seas and nights filled with restorative slumber.

It is common to assume that seeking help is a sign of weakness, but this couldn't be further from the truth. Engaging with dietitians, therapists, counselors, or physicians is an act of profound courage. It's the testament of a warrior willing to enlist allies for battles that require coalitions rather than solitary fighters.

Sometimes, you might feel that you're navigating your wellness journey with a compass perpetually spinning, unable to find true north. Hormonal imbalances, medical conditions, or life's transitions can scramble your internal signals. A doctor or an endocrinologist can be the one to calm the spin, offering clarity amidst confusion and charting a course back to equilibrium.

There are also instances when the mirror becomes an adversary, reflecting back a visage weighed down by societal expectations and pressure. In such moments, a psychologist or a body image consultant can help you to recognize your inherent value, teaching you to gaze upon your reflection with kindness and acceptance, rather than critique and dissatisfaction.

In your pursuit of a sustainable lifestyle, when the clamor of contradictory diet advice rings in your ears, a nutritionist can help you find the melody amid the noise. Their expertise can harmonize the information, providing a sound score to which you can tailor your eating habits, attuned perfectly to the symphony of your body's needs.

Turning the pages of your wellness story might reveal chapters filled with familial health conditions that lurk in your genetic narrative. Here, a genetic counselor can guide you through the complexities of inheritance, allowing you to make informed decisions that are proactive rather than reactive—preparing defenses before the specters of hereditary issues arise at your door.

Perhaps your enthusiasm for fitness has been crippled by injury, leaving you hesitant to engage in previously joyous activities. Physical therapists stand at the ready, equipped with their expertise in human kinetics, to rehabilitate not only your body but also your confidence, coaxing you back into the dance of movement without fear.

And as you journey on, be comforted by the thought that these beacons—the counselors, dietitians, doctors, psychologists, and trainers—are not mere sentinels dotting the path: they are fellow journeyers. They walk alongside you, offering their lanterns to illuminate your steps, sharing their compasses to point out the north star of your ambition on the nights where it seems most dim.

So when you find yourself questioning if now is the moment to seek help, trust your intuition as you would trust the sea to know its tides. When the current of your wellness journey tugs insistently, signaling that it's time for guidance, relinquish the helm ever so slightly.

Chapter 9:
The Role of Self-Compassion in Weight Loss

In the labyrinthine journey of weight loss, a most intimate ally we find in the art of self-compassion emerges as an unexpected guardian against the shadowlands of discouragement. As we peel back the curtains of strict self-discipline, this chapter unfurls the gentle embrace of accepting oneself amid the tumultuous tides of progress and setbacks. It's not simply about praising the pounds shed; it's about weaving a tapestry of kindness within one's own heart, for how can one nourish the body without first nurturing the soul? When the path ahead seems steep, or a stumble leaves you weary, self-compassion becomes the soothing balm that quiets the harsh critic within. As indulgent as a sunrise that warms the chilled dawn, acknowledging one's efforts, however small, lights the way towards sustainable change. Here, you will discover self-compassion as not a mere concept, but an essential traveler's companion on your quest for wellness. It's about transforming the inner dialogue from a tyrant's scorn to a mentor's cheer, allowing you to rise from the ashes of old habits with resilience and grace. With each chapter of your journey, remember this simple truth: the heart that learns to forgive itself is the very one that beats strongest under the sun of adversity.

Rethinking Perfection: Embrace Progress, Not Perfection

In the quest for weight loss and overall well-being, we often find ourselves ensnared by the illusive allure of perfection. The myriad of glossy magazine covers and seemingly flawless representations of health can skew our perceptions. Yet, it's paramount to shift our focus from the pursuit of an unattainable ideal to the embrace of progress.

Perfection is not just elusive; it's a mirage. Striving for absolute perfection can lead to a detrimental cycle of guilt and self-reproach when the unavoidable human slips occur. Isn't it wiser, then, to celebrate each step forward, no matter how small it may appear? Progress, after all, is a journey of incremental steps.

To progress is to move steadily forward, to learn from setbacks rather than being derailed by them. During a weight loss journey, it's crucial to recognize that lapses in diet or hiccups in an exercise routine are not failures but rather opportunities for learning and growth.

Could there be beauty in the struggle, in the unvarnished reality of effort and persistence? When we shed the weight of seeking perfection, we free ourselves to be more creative, more flexible, and to enjoy the process more fully. Self-compassion then becomes our ally, patting us on the back for our hard-won victories and whispering encouragement when the road becomes steep.

Imagine a balancing scale, with perfection on one end and progress on the other. The pursuit of perfection often tilts us into a sense of imbalance, where nothing seems quite good enough. Yet, as we tip the scales towards progress, balance is restored, and wellness in both body and mind becomes more attainable.

Self-compassion during weight loss means speaking to oneself as one would to a dear friend. Would we berate a friend for not reaching perfection, or would we emphasize their growth and cheer them on? This gentler, kinder approach to our own health journey not only fosters a healthier self-image but can lead to more sustainable change.

There's a rhythm to riding the waves of progress—between steady advancements and brief plateaus, the dance goes on. Taking time to reflect on how far one has come rather than how far one has yet to go can be a powerful motivator. This reflection can fuel the courage required to press on, step by step, toward wellness goals.

It's been shown that individuals who practice self-compassion are more likely to dust themselves off and try again after a setback. They're the resilient ones who understand that the path isn't always smooth and that detours don't lead to dead ends, but to lessons that strengthen resolve.

The beauty of emphasizing progress over perfection lies in the space it creates for triumphs that are not tied to a scale or a dietary checklist. These triumphs include the joyous realization of stronger self-discipline, the discovery of one's inner strength, and the gradual building of a healthier lifestyle that feels less like chastisement and more like nurturing.

Consider how an artist might craft a sculpture. It's not the finished figure that solely defines its worth, but the artist's ability to see potential in a block of marble and to chip away dutifully, fully absorbed in every stroke of the chisel. Weight loss, similarly, is a form of artistry applied to the self. It's in the daily discipline, the small choices, and the repeated efforts where true transformation takes shape.

Furthermore, it is crucial to identify how perfectionism can manifest as a barrier. It can masquerade as procrastination, waiting for the perfect day to start, or as an immutable routine that leaves no room for life's spontaneity. Embracing imperfection, on the other hand, can help build resilience against these sneaky impediments.

Adopting a mindset of growth rather than perfection allows us to revel in the journey. Each meal is not a test of self-worth but an occasion to choose well and to learn. Every workout becomes less about burning calories and more about celebrating movement and the body's capability.

It's also important to note that embracing progress does not mean abandoning standards or settling for mediocrity. It means setting realistic, achievable goals and recognizing that the path to reaching them is as important as the goals themselves. Strive for excellence, certainly, but let that striving be laced with patience and understanding.

Let us, therefore, approach weight loss with a renewed sense of purpose—one that values progress, cheers the small victories, and knows that wellness is a tapestry woven through time, effort, and the gentle art of self-compassion. It becomes not a struggle for a perfect body but a journey towards a healthier and more fulfilled self.

Whether one is taking the first step or the hundredth, the spirit of progress hums a tune of encouragement. Let that tune be your anthem, the background music to a life lived not in the shadow of perfection, but in the warm light of continuous growth and self-improvement. That, my friends, is the heart of true wellness.

Celebrating Milestones: Recognize and Reward Yourself

The odyssey of weight loss is laden with victories both grand and minute, each deserving its own herald. It is within the grand tapestry of self-compassion that the significance of celebrating milestones takes on a radiant hue. Let's unfurl the ways and whys behind marking your progress with joy and personal accolades.

Imagine: amidst the tumult of daily life, you've set your intentions, you've maintained discipline, and you've seen results, however modest. It's essential not to bypass these moments, as it's these very triumphs that build a resilient and sustained journey towards wellness. To recognize one's own progress is to anchor oneself in a state of gratitude and motivation.

Weight loss is no meager feat; it's a testament to one's dedication and fortitude. When you hit a milestone, big or small, pause and reflect. It's a juncture to look back at the road trodden and to relish the fruits of your labor.

Rewards needn't always be grandiose or material. Sometimes, a private moment to jot down the sensations and emotions tied to your accomplishments in a journal serves as a powerful reminder of your path and progress. Inscribe your journey so that on days when the will wanes, these recorded triumphs can reignite the spark of commitment.

Consider, also, the impact of sharing your milestones with others. Turning to your tribe—a cornerstone of any sustainable wellness journey—you'll find cheerleaders eager to extol your every step. Their words of encouragement weave into the tapestry of your accomplishments, adding texture and color.

That said, tangible rewards have a charm of their own. Treating yourself to a much-desired book, a serene spa day, or perhaps an enchanting evening at the theater, can act as an external representation of your internal growth. These moments of indulgence are not just frivolities; they are rites of passage, marking the transformation within.

Let us not overlook the simple yet satiating reward of nourishment. Preparing a delectable meal that harmonizes with your nutritional goals, brimming with color and flavor, serves as both a celebration and a reinforcement of mindful eating practices.

When you've crossed a particularly challenging threshold, or perhaps reached a halfway mark, why not invest in a tangible symbol that you can wear or keep close—a talisman to remind you of your journey every day. It could be a piece of jewelry, a small token for your pocket, or a piece of art for your sanctuary.

Additionally, upgrading your tools of transformation, such as a new pair of running shoes or a state-of-the-art blender, doubles as both reward and reinvestment into your health and wellness journey. These are not mere possessions; they are the armamentarium for your ongoing battle and victory over the old self.

Do not underestimate the power of experiences as rewards. Maybe it's a workshop or a class you've had your eye on—something that enhances your life and expands your horizons while aligning with your wellness vision. Education and experiences blend together as they mold your new self, sculpting the visage of the person you are becoming.

It's also worthwhile to align your rewards with your long-term wellness goals. If reaching a certain milestone means you're that much closer to a fitter lifestyle, perhaps a biking adventure or a hike in nature would be emblematic of your progress. Celebrate within the realm of your new lifestyle to foster a sense of unity with your ambitions.

Remember that these celebrations are not a full stop, but rather commas in the ongoing sentence of your wellness narrative. Each marks a breath, a moment to collect oneself before continuing on. They serve as amiable companions and gentle motivators along this winding path you tread.

It's crucial to tailor your rewards to be personally meaningful. What tugs at the heartstrings for one may not move another. Tune into your desires and passions when choosing how to commemorate your milestones. Let your rewards be a mirror reflecting your individuality and accentuating your unique journey.

As you recognize and reward yourself, be mindful not to let celebrations serve as mere intermissions between bouts of rigid discipline. Allow them to be part of the fabric of your new lifestyle, seamlessly integrated and equally important as your hard work and perseverance.

Finally, the practice of celebrating milestones in itself fosters a relationship with self-compassion. It's a means to gently remind ourselves that we are not just end-goals or outcomes, but evolving beings worthy of praise at every step. So, as you pave your path toward wellness, let every milestone be a beacon that lights your way, and each reward a cherished chapter in your ever-unfolding story of health and self-discovery.

Chapter 10:
The Science of Metabolism and Weight Control

Turning the page on our empowering narrative, we delve into the intricate dance of metabolism and weight, where every calorie and every step waltz in the ballroom of our bodies with scientific precision. This chapter unfurls the tapestry of metabolism, that enigmatic maestro commanding the ebb and flow of energy conversion within us. Let's illuminate the hidden alcoves of this biological machinery, exploring how it can be gently coaxed to whirl in harmonious tandem with our weight control endeavors. We'll traverse the landscape of our metabolic rate—the steady hum of calorie burning—and observe how the passage of time might cause it to shift rhythm. With a blend of gentle persuasion and vivid imagery, we'll escort you toward a deeper understanding, aiming to equip you with the keys of knowledge that can unlock the doors to a balanced and sustainable control of weight. Remember, it's a harmonious interplay of elements in which you are both the conductor and the orchestra. Herein lies the alchemy that transforms the pangs of hunger and the sweat of exertion into the gold of well-being and fitness.

Understanding Your Metabolic Rate

Slip with me, if you will, into the fascinating world of metabolic mysteries. It's a realm where every calorie counts, but not all calories are created equal. Just as a maestro conducts an orchestra, your metabolic rate sets the tempo for your body's energy consumption. It's the measure of how fast your body burns calories. The faster the metabolism, the more energetic the symphony. Standing as the cornerstone of our wellness architecture, understanding it is a quest well worth embarking on.

Picture your metabolism as a hearth. In this hearth, the fires need to be tended—fuel added periodically, oxygen supplied, and the embers raked to encourage a vibrant flame. In a similar light, your metabolic rate can be fueled and nurtured, influenced by diverse factors like genetics, muscle mass, and even the type of foods you consume. Grasping the inner workings of this metabolic blaze is the first step towards mastering the art of weight control.

The concept of basal metabolic rate (BMR) is crucial. It's the number of calories your body requires at rest to maintain vital functions—like your heart beating, lungs breathing, and cells renewing. Your BMR consumes a sizable chunk of your daily calorie expenditure, which is an intriguing piece of trivia and a pivotal health detail. However, it's not just a matter of intrinsic bodily functions; BMR varies from person to person, influenced by age, gender, size, and body composition.

Now, step beyond BMR, and we encounter the total daily energy expenditure (TDEE)—the overall calories you burn in a day, which includes all your activities, from the minute you rise until you retire at night. If you're aiming to lose weight, it's your TDEE that most dieticians will point you towards. After all, to lose weight, one must consume fewer calories than what's burned—creating what's known as a 'caloric deficit'.

Here's something thought-provoking—lean muscle mass matters. Muscle tissue burns more calories at rest compared to fat tissue. This fact alone can spur a shift in one's approach to weight loss. Forging an alliance with strength training could turn out to be a resilient partner in your quest for fitness, subtly sculpting your body into a more efficient calorie-burning machine, even amidst the serenity of slumber.

What we eat also plays a delicate dance with our metabolism. Some foods, armed with a thermal effect, can slightly accelerate this metabolic pace. Spicy foods, protein-rich meals, and green tea—these are but a few of the culinary crusaders that can aid this process. It's a small edge, certainly, but an edge nonetheless. Weight management, as we shall see, is an affair that reaches beyond mere calorie counting.

Chronic stress, our unseen adversary, can throw our metabolic rate into disarray. When stress enters the scene, it brings cortisol—often referred to as the stress hormone. Cortisol can promote fat storage, particularly around the midsection, and slow down the metabolism. It could be said that taming the tempest of stress is as important for metabolic health as it is for mental well-being.

As we sit at the table of discussions on metabolism, we cannot sidestep the role of hormones. Thyroid hormones, for instance, are instrumental in orchestrating our metabolic rhythm. An imbalance in these hormones can lead to fluctuations in weight. Hypothyroidism—a condition of an underactive thyroid—can decelerate the metabolic rate, often culminating in weight gain.

Another intriguing dynamic is how our metabolic rate adjusts as part of a response to weight loss. Sometimes, in its quest to maintain equilibrium, the body will slow down the metabolism to conserve energy—this is a phenomenon known as adaptive thermogenesis. It's the body's survival mechanism, one that was perhaps handy in times of yore, when food scarcity was a genuine concern, but now serves as a modern-day hurdle in weight loss ventures.

Don't let this discourage you, though. Instead, let it fortify your resolve with knowledge and strategy. One such approach is to combine aerobic activity with resistance training. Aerobic activity, by burning a high number of calories, can chip away at weight, while resistance training maintains and potentially builds muscle mass to support a robust metabolic rate.

Timing can also impact your metabolic rate. Meal frequency, the long-debated character in our nutritional novel, might have a role in metabolic fluctuations. Some argue that smaller, frequent meals can keep the metabolic engine humming along. Yet, others champion intermittent fasting as a means to aid metabolic health. The jury may still be out, but it's a conversation worth having with one's own body—listening to its cues and judging what fuels it best.

Hydration, the source of life itself, mustn't be ignored. Even mild dehydration can dampen your metabolic rate. Like a stream that flows more vigorously after a fresh rain, your metabolism too can be enlivened with ample hydration. It's a simple act—a glass of water—but its repercussions on metabolic health and weight management are profound.

Finally, let's talk about temperatures. Believe it or not, the body burns more calories when it has to regulate its temperature—either in the cold, as it works to keep warm, or in heat as it cools down. This doesn't suggest drastic measures, like relocating to a frigid climate or taking ice baths, but it opens up a fascinating arena in metabolic science: the potential of temperature to influence calorie burn.

All these threads we've spun—muscle mass, food choices, hormones, physical activity, and more—they weave together into the tapestry of our metabolic rate. Understanding this interconnected nature is a powerful tool in your arsenal for health and wellness.

As we linger at the edge of the rich panorama that is metabolism and weight control, let's remember that knowledge is the greatest architect of change. With the secrets of our metabolic rate in our grasp, we're empowered to craft a more fine-tuned approach to wellness. It calls for patience, curiosity, and an open mind, as each body sings its unique metabolic aria. Now, equipped with the key to decode your metabolic rhythm, you're better poised to harmonize your health symphony to your desired tune.

Adapting for Age: Metabolism Over Time

As the hands of time steadily march forward, it is an indisputable truth that our bodies mature along a concurrent path, winding and complex—a journey that invariably brings about change in our complex biological machinery. Among these changes, metabolism, that bewilderingly intricate dance of chemical reactions, keeps an enigmatic tempo, slowing with the passing years. Understanding this natural evolution isn't just an exercise in biological curiosity; it's paramount to tailoring our health strategies as we progress through life's rich tapestry.

When we are young, lithe, and spirited, our bodies are metabolic marvels, efficiently converting food we consume into the energy that fuels us. But lo and behold, as we cross the threshold beyond our twenties, a subtle shift tends to stir. The once-radiant flame of youthful metabolism—capable of incinerating a late-night feast to mere embers by morning—begins its inevitable wane, typically descending by a rate some dare to quantify; a decrement of approximately 1-2% per decade.

This metabolic shift isn't a furtive thief in the night, stealing away our vitality without warning. It's a gradual transition, affected by shifts in muscle mass and hormonal changes amongst many other factors. An awareness and understanding of this change can be an ally in our quest for health and wellness—nay, in our defiance of time's relentless march.

For many, the alarm bells sound at the mention of muscle mass reduction—a primary catalyst in the slowing of metabolic rates. Muscle—an avid consumer of energy, even in repose—plays a vital role. As their abundance ebbs, so too does our body's innate ability to torch calories without breaking a sweat. Thus, the weight that once posed no issue slowly but assertively stakes its claim around waists and hips, until we either challenge it, or accept it as an unwelcome guest.

How, then, can one parry the blows of advancing age to one's metabolic fortune? Strength training, my friends, extends an olive branch. Engage in the purposeful sculpting and fortification of your musculature, and you shall find a comrade in the struggle against metabolic slowdown. Lifting weights, resistance bands, or even one's own body weight can forge the muscle needed to stoke the metabolic fires.

Yet, muscle isn't the sole determinant of one's metabolic fate; hormones play their own capricious games. Thyroid function, estrogen, testosterone—all morph with the accumulating annals of our personal history, impacting metabolism. Ah, but we are not mere spectators in this game! Careful attention to diet, exercise, and even consultation with medical experts can mitigate these hormonal roller coasters, allowing us to maintain a semblance of metabolic grace.

What's more, the body's insulin sensitivity—a key player in how effectively it uses glucose—also ebbs with age. A diet rich in whole foods, ample fiber, and judicious portions can help navigate these choppy glucose waters. Ensuring the body's cells respond well to insulin is like engaging in a delicate, yet deeply consequential ballet with our blood sugar levels.

Let's consider also the oft-overlooked aspects of metabolism that are digestive health and gut flora. As twilight encroaches upon one's years, digestive enzymes—trustworthy facilitators of nutrient absorption—can become less abundant. A diet replete with probiotics and foods that aid digestion becomes a clarion call for those seeking metabolic equilibrium.

And what of our eating patterns, those rhythmic rituals we enact daily? Intermittent fasting emerges as a muse for some, offering not only weight management but improved metabolic variables. This symphony of eating and fasting can recalibrate our metabolic mechanisms, helping counteract the slow-down that age so wistfully introduces.

Nor should we neglect the elixir of life itself: water. Adequate hydration can facilitate a more effervescent metabolism. Yet with age, our senses often betray us, dulling thirst, leaving us oblivious to the needs of our cells. Let it be known that ensuring a regular intake of water is a simple yet effective step toward maintaining metabolic vibrancy.

Considering sleep, that sweet surrender to nightly restoration, we uncover its critical role in metabolic health. Poor or insufficient sleep can beget a sluggish metabolism. Thus, prioritizing a restful, regular sleep schedule becomes an essential strategy in the battle to preserve our metabolic prowess.

Stress, too, wields a double-edged sword, its blade sharpened with cortisol—a hormone that, in excess, whispers seductively to the body to store fat, particularly around the midsection. Strategies to manage stress, whether through meditation, deep breathing, or leisure activities, are paramount in safeguarding the metabolism from this insidious foe.

Yet, let us not fall prey to fatalism, assuming that age's toll on metabolism is a curse we must simply endure. Individual variance is a beacon of hope, a reminder that the proverbial "metabolic clock" doesn't tick uniformly for all. Some may find themselves blessed with a fiery metabolism well into their later years, a testament to genetics, lifestyle, and perhaps a sprinkle of serendipity.

And so, as the chapters of our lives unfurl, we must adapt our approach with agility and finesse. Regular metabolic check-ups, an attentive eye on body composition, and a willingness to reshape our habits with the wisdom of experience can serve us well in this odyssey. The pursuit of maintaining a balanced metabolism, despite the encroachment of time, is not only about weight control—it's about sustaining the vivacious spirit within that yearns for lifelong health and vitality.

As with all things in this intricate dance of life, a holistic view of one's health is necessary. A sound metabolism is but one note in the symphony of a well-lived life, resonating in harmony with other aspects of wellness covered throughout this book. Adapt we must, as change is the only constant, to keep ourselves in tune with the melody of life—and weight management is but one measure in our opus of existence.

Chapter 11:
Integrative Approaches to Weight Loss

As we turn the page to a fresh chapter, we find a treasury of wisdom on weight loss that reaches far beyond the familiar land of diets and dumbbells. In the grand tapestry of health, it's time to weave in the golden threads of holistic practices that paint a more comprehensive picture of well-being. Imagine a symphony where each note represents a unique habit or remedy, and together they create a harmonious melody of weight management. Yes, think green smoothies armed with the might of micronutrients and yoga poses that stretch the body as well as the soul. Here's where we explore how the subtle alchemy of proper supplementation, when paired with physical endeavors, can optimize the very essence of your body's constitution. In this realm, the adage that 'you are what you eat' expands to 'you are the lifestyle you lead', merging modern insights with timeless traditions, coaxing the scale to benevolently tip in our favor without the discord of deprivation.

Holistic Health Practices: Beyond the Basics

Embarking on a comprehensive wellness journey often begins with the familiar pillars of health - nutrition, exercise, sleep, and psychological well-being. But the realm of holistic health broadens the spectrum, ushering in a world where balance and sustainability are not merely cogs in the weight loss machine, but rather vital components that permeate every facet of living vibrantly. Here, we explore the art and science of augmenting your integrative approaches to weight loss with practices that extend beyond the basic tenets.

One often overlooked element of a holistic health paradigm is the interplay of natural elements with our well-being. The sun, air, and earth are allies in our quest for health; turning one's face to bask in the sun's rays is not mere indulgence but a source of vitamin D, essential for bone health and metabolic function. Outdoor exercise marries the benefits of physical activity with fresh air and a connection to nature, enhancing both respiratory function and mental clarity.

Water, too, plays a critical role. Hydration goes beyond simply quenching thirst - it's a cornerstone for metabolic processes and aids in detoxification. When the body is well-hydrated, it's like a stream flowing briskly, as opposed to a stagnant pond. Furthermore, practices like hydrotherapy, which might include contrasts of hot and cold water, can invigorate the system and promote better circulation.

The gut is dubbed the second brain for a reason, and nurturing gut health is a key player in holistic wellness. Probiotics, prebiotics, and a diet rich in varied fibers support a flourishing microbiome, which in turn influences everything from mood to immune function. Digestion is more than breaking down food; it's about assimilating nutrients and expelling what doesn't serve us, both physically and metaphorically.

Then there is the vast universe of herbal supplements, remedies steeped in tradition and supported by modern research. While not all herbs are created equal, and care must be taken to understand their properties and potential interactions, many offer support for metabolism, stress, sleep, and overall vitality. Plants such as ashwagandha for stress, green tea for metabolic boost, and chamomile for relaxation integrate seamlessly into a diet and underscore nature's bounty.

Above diet and supplements lies the powerful yet intangible world of energy. Modalities such as Reiki, qi gong, and acupuncture may seem enigmatic, tapping into unseen forces of life energy, or 'qi', to promote harmony and healing. While the mechanisms may elude the grasp of conventional science, many find solace and tangible benefits in these practices, echoing millennia of holistic traditions.

Breath, the most fundamental of life's rhythms, is another formidable tool. Breathwork practices, ranging from the simplicity of deep diaphragmatic breathing to the complexities of pranayama in yoga, offer a profound way to modulate the nervous system. In the ebb and flow of inhale and exhale lies the potential to calm or energize, to detoxify and to center. It's a direct line to the body's physiological control panel, one breath at a time.

Speaking of yoga, this ancient practice embodies holistic philosophy. With poses (asanas) to strengthen and stretch, and meditative components to soothe the mind, yoga is a full-spectrum approach to wellness. Weight loss may be a welcome side effect, yet the main prize is the unity of mind, body, and spirit.

Never forget the touch. Therapeutic massage and bodywork release muscle tension, improve circulation, and can even facilitate emotional release. In an age of screens and distance, the power of human touch has never seemed more sacred, nor more essential to holistic health.

Moving on from the tangible to the intangible, let's consider sound and its healing properties. Sound therapy, whether through music, singing bowls, or the human voice, can shift mood, induce relaxation, and possibly even improve cellular function. The vibrations we introduce into our environment, and thus into ourselves, matter immensely.

Light exposure also plays a significant role. The rhythms of our body are tied to the cycles of natural light, influencing sleep and hormones like melatonin and cortisol. Using tools like light therapy to mimic natural light patterns can be especially beneficial in managing energy levels and circadian rhythm.

To round out the spectrum of holistic health, one must consider the less tangible aspects of our existence - our social bonds, purpose, and joy. Engaging in community, fulfilling work, and hobbies that light a spark within are not mere luxuries but foundational to our well-being. They shape our world from the inside out, offering contentment that cannot be measured in pounds and inches, but rather in satisfaction and vitality.

Let us also acknowledge the spirituality that lies at the heart of holistic health. Regardless of one's personal beliefs, recognizing something greater than ourselves provides a framework for understanding our place in the tapestry of life. It lends perspective to our health and wellness journey, providing both humility and a sense of connection.

Finally, remember, the path to holistic health is not linear, nor is it the same for every individual. It requires tuning in - to your body, to nature, and to the silent whispers of your intuition. It's a dance of trial and learning, of respecting ancient wisdom while heeding the advice of modern science.

These practices, beyond the basics of diet and exercise, forge a more profound relationship with well-being. They offer a tapestry of approaches that honor the complexities of the human experience and lend credence to the notion that weight management is but one piece of the greater mosaic of health. May you explore these vistas with openness and find the unique concoction of practices that resonate with your body, your mind, and your spirit.

Supplementing Your Diet: When to Consider Vitamins and Minerals

In the spirited dance of weight loss, where diet and exercise lead, the ever-attentive partners of vitamins and minerals often glide unnoticed in the background. Yet, their role in orchestrating the symphony of wellness cannot be understated. While whole foods should always be the prima ballerinas of your dietary stage, sometimes the encores of life's demands can leave gaps in nutrition. This is where dietary supplements pirouette in, providing targeted support to ensure that your body's needs are seamlessly met.

Embarking on the journey of weight loss, you may find many roads, yet not all are paved with the necessary sustenance. It's here that you might ponder the role of that bottled array of vitamins and minerally endowed concoctions. To supplement or not to supplement, that might be the question weighing as heavily on your mind as the pounds you aim to shed.

One may be inclined to think that a well-balanced diet would suffice, and for many, it does. However, in our helter-skelter world, with its fast pace and faster foods, achieving that balance is akin to a tightrope walk in a tempest. Herein lies the conundrum: even the most intentional eaters among us can find themselves beset by nutritional deficits, whispering the siren call for additional health harbors.

Toying with the idea of supplementation should not be done with a cavalier heart; instead, let us move forward with judicious minds. Assess your diet carefully; what does it contain, and equally important, what might it lack? Certain populations are more susceptible to deficiencies—such as pregnant individuals, the elderly, or those with specific dietary restrictions—which makes the case for dietary supplements more compelling.

Witness the mighty Vitamin D—so often lacking, especially in those who shun the sun or live in climes less kissed by its rays. This stalwart guardian of bone health and immune function often falls short in our intakes, urging many experts to whisper of its necessity in hushed, yet urgent tones.

Iron, too, must enter this conversation, stepping forward with the gravitas befitting its crucial role in combatting tiredness and fatigue—common villains in the narrative of weight loss. Particular attention to iron is warranted for those amongst us on a vegetarian or vegan path, or for women with heavier menstrual cycles.

And who can forget the B vitamins—those conductors of energy production within the body? They ensure our cells are well-fueled and our engines are running at peak performance. A deficiency might manifest as the lethargy that so often derails the well-intentioned dieter from their track.

Then there's Omega-3 fatty acids, usually headlining seafood extravaganzas but also playing cameo roles in flaxseeds and walnuts. They oil the cogs of our cardiovascular system and douse the inflammatory fires within. For those who rarely partake in Neptune's bounty, supplementation can bridge an expansive gap.

Fiber, albeit not a vitamin or mineral, deserves a courteous nod for its role in satiety and digestive health. Those navigating the weight loss maze without enough fiber often find themselves hungry and harried, making a supplementary boost worth considering.

Calcium joins the soiree, arm-in-arm with Vitamin D, to bolster bones and encourage their longevity. While dairy often dons the cape of calcium heroism, those donning the attire of dietary restrictions may find themselves in need of a supplemental sidekick.

While consideration of these supplements is wise, caution should be your watchword. Excess can be as precarious as scarcity, and the principle of moderation should be the lighthouse guiding you through the murky waters of choice.

Remember that dietary supplements are not vindicated actors on the stage of regulation; the oversight is less stringent, making your role in selecting high-quality supplements more critical. Choose reputable brands, those whose transparency is not shrouded in mystery, and whose products have stood the test of scientific scrutiny.

Consultation with healthcare professionals can turn the muddled cacophony of supplementation options into a harmonious melody. A dietitian or nutritionist's wisdom, flowing as freely as the pen of a seasoned scribe, can direct you to the nutritional notes that will complement your dietary symphony.

In moments of consideration for dietary augmentation, do not bow to the tyranny of trends or the pressure of peers. Your body, a temple uniquely yours, has bespoke needs and iIndividualized rhythms, and what works for one may not work for another. Tune into your body's subtle signals—its whispers of fatigue, its aches, and its highs—and let these guide your hand when reaching for supplementation.

As the curtain falls on this chapter, we're reminded that supplementation is not the panacea for all our ills, but a potential co-star in the grand production of wellness. It can't replace the solid foundations of a balanced diet and active lifestyle. However, when used discerningly, vitamins and minerals can help fill the gaps, ensuring the body is well-nourished to meet the demands of weight loss and overall health. Let this, then, be your guiding star—a balanced approach where supplementation complements, not overshadows, the staples of your well-curated dietary repertoire.

Chapter 12:
Staying Motivated and Maintaining Progress

In the melodious narrative of our health and wellness odyssey, maintaining the symphony of motivation amidst the cacophony of life's distractions is a quest that requires both resilience and finesse. Like the ebb and flow of an enigmatic river, the waters of progress and motivation can surge with vivacity or dwindle to a sluggish stream. Yet fear not, for within these pages lie the very essence of perpetual motion and the secrets to fueling the inner flame that propels us forward. How might one summon the strength to persevere when the path seems shrouded in mist? One finds fuel in a tapestry woven from the golden threads of visualization, where the mind's eye holds a vision so radiant, it illuminates the steps ahead. When barriers rise like formidable specters, strategies not unlike the measured strokes of an artist's brush, paint a pathway around, over, or through the seemingly insurmountable. One's journey is not simply a matter of crossing distances measured in pounds or inches, but of nurturing the embers of determination that warm the spirit even in the chill of challenge. Thus equipped, the voyage towards wellness is not a tale of grim endurance, but one of vibrant evolution, a story written not with ink, but with the very essence of human fortitude.

Visualization and Affirmations: Harnessing the Power of the Mind

Motivation is a fickle friend; it visits us in a flourish at the dawn of our wellness journey and yet can scamper away like a phantom in the night when we most yearn for its presence. To lure it back into our grasp and maintain the momentum of progress, we must turn to the less tangible, oft-misunderstood tools at our disposal: visualization and affirmations. These are the instruments of the mind that can transform our internal landscape as surely as a skilled gardener tends to their flora.

Imagine if you will, the power lying dormant within your own thoughts. To visualize is to paint the canvas of your mind with the intricate details of your desired reality. It's to see the svelte figure in the mirror, to feel the pulse of robust health beating through your veins, to hear the whispers of praise from loved ones and feel a surge of pride swell within your chest. This mental practice is not mere daydreaming—it's a focused rehearsal for reality.

Affirmations, those small, seemingly innocuous phrases we repeat to ourselves, are akin to the strokes of a brush on the aforementioned canvas. With each utterance, you're chiseling away at the old sculptures of self-doubt and reshaping them into pillars of self-belief. "I am capable", "I am worthy", "I am progressing", they echo in the inner sanctum of your being, resonating with the frequency of truth.

For the skeptics who might consider such exercises frivolous or indulgent, let's remember that our brain's reticular activating system (RAS), that vigilant sentry, is proficient in identifying and prioritizing information aligned with our focus. When we immerse ourselves in the vivid details of our visualization, when we saturate our self-speak with affirmations, we're essentially programming our RAS to spotlight opportunities and resources that propel us towards our aspirations.

It is quite simple to begin this journey of the mind. Find a quiet corner, a personal sanctuary, where you can be undisturbed. Close your eyes and breathe deeply. Start to conjure the vision of your healthiest self. What are you doing? How do you feel? Who is with you? Engage all senses to the fullest extent, crafting a scenario so tangible you can almost reach out and touch it.

As important as the visions are the words we weave into our daily narrative. A daily affirmation ritual can be as straightforward as repeating your chosen mantras while brushing your teeth or during those first waking moments. It's essential to select affirmations that resonate on a personal level, are positively framed, and stated in the present tense. This present-focus tricks the mind into working towards alignment with these affirmations—cultivating a fertile ground for growth.

Combined, visualization and affirmations forge a formidable bond. Just as a gardener imagines the future blossoms while planting seeds, you must envision your success and speak it into existence. Both practices engage the subconscious, which is a powerful influencer of our actions and reactions. They create a loop of positivity that can sustain motivation through the driest spells.

Consider the story of an athlete preparing for a significant race. They envision themselves breaking through the tape, feeling the rubbery track underfoot, hearing the roar of the crowd. They tell themselves time and again, "I am swift, I am strong, I endure." As they train, this mental blueprint guides their efforts, infusing their muscles with purpose and tenacity. So too must the individual seeking wellness recalibrate their mindset with these tools.

Furthermore, the science of neuroplasticity tells us that our brains are not the rigid structures we once believed them to be; they are pliable, ever-changing landscapes. Each time we engage in visualization or affirmations, we are etching new pathways, constructing new bridges, and fostering a network of brain signals that champion our wellness goals.

But let us be clear, this is not about wishful thinking or magical outcomes derived from thin air. No, this is about the deliberate crafting of internal narratives that shape external behaviors. When the instinct is to retreat, it is the mental rehearsal that whispers, "advance." When the world tells you it's too late, or too hard, your affirmations insist, "It's my time, and I am capable."

Visualizations and affirmations are not solitary practices; they are complemented by action. They are the undercurrent propelling you towards sensible eating, towards embracing exercise—even when it's challenging, towards choosing rest and recovery over relentless strain. They move you past temporary stagnation and into the realms of incremental triumphs.

Think of it as sculpting clay. Each day you mold a little more, sometimes reshaping entire sections, other times refining delicate details. The clay is your habits, your choices, your mindset, and your hands are guided by the clarity of your vision and the cadence of your affirmations.

It's also about authenticity in your vision and affirmations. A borrowed dream or a mantra that doesn't speak your truth will feel hollow, like a poorly fitted garment. Craft them as you would craft a living thing—with care, with sincerity, and with patience. It's this authenticity that fuels the fire of motivation and keeps the hearth of progress alight.

As you continue along your wellness journey, remember that visualization and affirmations are vital companions. They are reflections of your resilience, your tenacity, and your unwavering commitment to health and wellness. They are the gentle guardians that keep your motivations kindled, your actions aligned, and your progress ever onward.

And so, with the mind as both the canvas and the brush, let us wield visualization and affirmations as the skilled artists of our health and wellness that we are. Let us turn the intangible into the tangible and shape the life we aspire to—one focused thought, one heartfelt affirmation at a time.

Overcoming Obstacles: Strategies to Keep Moving Forward

As we tread the path of health and wellness, our journey is punctuated by a series of hurdles and setbacks. Yet, it is through these challenges that our resolve is truly tested and our determination to push forward solidified. In the grand scheme of wellness, overcoming obstacles becomes an integral part of the narrative.

Firstly, when confronted with a barrier, the power of perspective cannot be understated. Viewing hurdles not as impenetrable walls but rather as opportunities to learn and grow can transform the nature of the challenge itself. It's a subtle shift in mindset, but a powerful one – for the person who embraces their obstacles is already on the path to overcoming them.

It's common to face periods where motivation wanes and progress seems to inch at a tortoise-like pace. During such times, reconnecting with the initial spark that ignited your wellness journey can reignite the dwindling flame. Reflect on your 'why' and let it be the beacon that guides you through the fog of discouragement.

There will be occasions when the well-intended plans for diet and exercise fall to the wayside, overwhelmed by the vagaries of life. It's crucial then to not dwell in self-reproach, but to gently and firmly guide oneself back on course. Forgiveness is a balm, allowing us to treat ourselves with kindness as we navigate back to our desired path.

Goal setting is another stalwart ally in the journey of wellness. Rather than lofty and distant objectives, crafting small, achievable goals allows for the sweet taste of success to be savored more frequently. These victories, however minor, build a scaffold of confidence, propelling us forward with renewed vigor.

Amidst the onslaught of daily demands, it's easy for one's wellness routine to be crowded out. Here, the art of time management steps in – an ally to be courted and mastered. By allocating specific slots in a day for activities that foster health and wellness, we carve out space for progress amidst the chaos.

Life invariably throws curveballs that disrupt our best-laid plans. When illness strikes or obligations pull us away from our routines, it's vital to adapt rather than capitulate. This may mean adjusting exercise intensity, modifying dietary choices, or seeking alternative methods to maintain mental health during trying times.

On the journey to weight loss and improved fitness, plateaus are a formidable yet common adversary. In the midst of stagnation, the key is to alter one's tactics – whether it's introducing new exercises, tweaking nutritional intake, or revaluating sleep and stress-management practices. Change spurs growth, and variety is the spice that rejuvenates a stale regimen.

A support system is not merely a luxury, but often a necessity in overcoming obstacles. Loneliness can erode resolve, so leaning on family, friends, or joining a community can offer the camaraderie and encouragement necessary to persist during tough times.

For moments when external support isn't enough, professional guidance may be the lifeline needed to cross treacherous waters. A nutritionist, personal trainer, or therapist can offer tailored advice and strategies to navigate through specific challenges, paving the way for continued progress.

Rejection of the all-or-nothing mentality also facilitates perseverance. Absolute perfection in diet or exercise routines is an unattainable myth that only leads to frustration. Celebrating incremental progress, no matter how insignificant it may seem, fosters a more forgiving and thus sustainable approach to wellness.

Stress, the insidious saboteur of health, must be managed with deft hands. Techniques like mindfulness, breathing exercises, and meditation not only assuage the stormy seas of stress but also enhance overall well-being - serving as tools to circumvent the barriers it creates.

At times when motivation is scarce, visualization and affirmations can serve as powerful catalysts. By vividly picturing the achievement of wellness goals and reinforcing them with positive self-talk, one can conjure the inner strength to overcome trials and tribulations.

When the shadow of a rut looms, mixing up routines can dispel the gloom. Trying new fitness classes, exploring different cuisines, or altering sleep schedules can provide a refreshing change of scenery for the mind and body, making the familiar journey novel once again.

Lastly, acknowledging that obstacles are an inherent part of any journey is fundamental. They are not indicators of failure, but rather milestones in the evolution of one's well-being. Embrace them, learn from them, and let them guide you to greater heights of health and happiness.

In the grand tapestry of wellness, every challenge transcended, every adversity navigated, enriches the fabric of our journey. With strategies to keep moving forward woven into our day-to-day lives, we not only overcome obstacles but also transform them into the threads that strengthen the resolve and enhance the beauty of our continuous quest for health and wellness.

Chapter 13:
Your Continuous Mindful Wellness Path

As our journey within these pages draws to a close, it is but a single step in the larger voyage toward your ever-evolving wellbeing. The tools and wisdom you've uncovered are the seeds from which your continual growth will spring. Keep in mind that your path to health and wellness holds the essence of ceaseless motion; it winds on with the grace of a river, ever forward, ever changing, enriched by every experience.

The wellness wheel has turned full circle, from your tastes and habits in nutrition to the wonders of movement through exercise. You've delved into the intricate dance of sleep and weight management, begun to untangle the psychology of eating, and envisioned the life wherein your wellness blooms fullest.

You've learned to see weight loss plateaus not as obstacles, but as invitations to refine your strategy, to know your body and mind more intimately. Stress, once an albatross around the neck of progress, is now understood as a thread in the fabric to be woven into strength through mindfulness.

The sacred connection between exercise and your mental state has been revealed, not merely as a concept, but as a felt, rhythmic pulse within your daily life. Mental fitness through mindful movement has become an essential part of your routine, something as natural as the rise and fall of your own breath.

Your explorations in nutrition culminated with not just a plate of balanced macros, but a plate filled with the vibrance of greens and the richness of a diversified diet. And community—the tribe you've built or are in the process of building—stands with you, not as onlookers, but as participants in this shared human pursuit of health and fulfillment.

The path is not absent of missteps or regression, and perfection was never the aim. Instead, it's about incremental victories, those quiet moments of self-kindness when you recognized your achievements and treated each milestone as a festival of your personal growth.

Understanding metabolism has offered insight into the "hows" and "whys" of your body's unique responses. Aging, once an adversary to your wellness goals, now sits beside you, sharing in the wisdom that comes with adapting gracefully over time.

Openness to integrative approaches has expanded your arsenal in the quest for wellness, with holistic practices and smart supplementation offering new avenues to explore what health means for you, in a body that is acknowledged as both biological and spiritual.

Maintaining motivation is an art as well as a science, drawing upon the profound power of visualization and affirmation. You've armed yourself with strategies and a steadfast resolve to thrive even when obstacles rise, as surely they will, against the horizon of your wellness journey.

So here you find yourself, at a threshold that is but another beginning. Your path stretches onward, not a straight line, but an ambling road, rich with turns and dips, peaks and valleys. It's a path best journeyed with eyes wide to the beauty of each step, and a heart ready to embrace change with gusto.

As you close this chapter, know that your path doesn't end here. It continues each day you draw breath. It persists in your choices, the small and silent as much as the grand. Each step is an inscription in the narrative of your life, each breath a testament to your willingness to live more fully, more mindfully, and with robust vigor.

Remember, your path is uniquely yours, woven from the threads of your individual experiences, challenges, dreams, and triumphs. While the guidance and strategies this book provides are the maps and compasses, you are the intrepid traveler, the cartographer charting the unexplored territories of your own being.

May each day find you with a heart more at peace and a mind attuned to the subtle yet powerful rhythms of a life lived with intention. For now, it's not farewell, but a gentle nod to the continuation of your passage, as you step forth, courageous and resolute, onto your continuous mindful wellness path.

And when you feel you need a confidant, remember the pages of this humble guide. They remain your steadfast companions, eternally poised to offer support, to remind you of your inner strength, and to rekindle the embers of motivation that lay ready to ignite within you. So, continue to nurture yourself as one would tend to a precious garden, for in that care, in that love for your well-being, lies the truest form of wealth one could ever hope to cultivate.

In the quiet reflection that follows, let gratitude wash over you for the strides you've made. With each day's end, a soft glow of contentment for the wellness journey you are crafting. Step by step, moment by moment, breathe by breathe—this is your continuous mindful wellness path.

Appendix A:
Tools and Resources for Further Exploration

As we've journeyed together through the complexities and possibilities of personal wellness and self-transformation, let us now arm ourselves with a treasure trove of resources that can act as a compass and map as we continue voyaging towards the pinnacles of health and fulfillment.

Recommended Reading and Websites

Embark upon a literary quest that will bolster knowledge and inspire action. Consider these beacons of wisdom:

The Mindful Diet - This tome provides insight into how mindfulness can unravel the intricate web of eating behaviors, spurring a transformative relationship with food.

Body Kindness – In this reflective volume, readers will discover the art of listening to one's body and the importance of self-compassion in health and wellness.

YogaJournal.com – An encyclopedic online repository of yoga wisdom, its pages are replete with sequences, meditations, and scholarly articles on the nexus of yoga and wellness.

ACE Fitness – Their digital hearth is an abundance of articles, workout plans, and expert advice on physical activity, from the rudimentary to the advanced.

Recipes for Healthy Living

Transform your kitchen into a laboratory of nourishment:

Explore the culinary landscapes with **MinimalistBaker.com**, where simplicity meets savor, offering recipes that can be crafted with ten ingredients or less.

Dive into the plant-based ocean of flavor with *Oh She Glows*, a cookbook brimming with recipes that cater to a wholesome life force.

Exercise Programs and Guides

Find the rhythm and pace that resonate with your soul, for movement is a symphony every body should serenade:

Fitness Blender – Discover a digital trove of exercises, where tailored programs meet the needs of beginners and seasoned athletes alike.

Darebee – A beacon for those who crave variety, Darebee offers a myriad of fitness challenges and workouts to keep one's physical quest fresh and invigorating.

It is within these pages, these URLs, and among the very steps of our continued strides where knowledge becomes our beacon and practice turns into progress. Whether your quest is for the body's strength, the mind's serenity, or a spirit filled with joy, may these tools and resources light your way as you forge your path in the life-affirming pursuit of health and wellness.

Recommended Reading and Websites

The quest for health and wellness is as much a journey of the mind as it is of the body. Empower your efforts further with wisdom and insights gleaned from a curated collection of reading materials and online resources. For those thirsty for knowledge and seeking companionship on their path to personal transformation, the lists that follow offer a veritable feast.

First to the treasure trove: books that offer profound insight into the harmonious balance of nutrition, fitness, and mental well-being. Titles such as "Eat, Move, Sleep" by Tom Rath can become trusted guides on the weaving path towards better health, encouraging you to see the inseparable link between the nourishment you take in, the vitality you nourish through movement, and the rejuvenation that only sleep can bestow.

For those who find solace in the narratives of others, memoirs like "It Was Me All Along" by Andie Mitchell share heartfelt journeys of weight loss and self-discovery that resonate with authenticity. They remind us that our struggles are surmountable and that our stories merit the telling.

On the forefront of scientific knowledge, "The Obesity Code" by Dr. Jason Fung peels back the layers of myth surrounding weight loss, providing readers with a robust understanding of the biological factors that dictate our body's responses. A most enlightening read, indeed, for those seeking explanation in lieu of exasperation.

Translating these insights to practical action, delve into trustworthy websites such as NutritionFacts.org or MyFitnessPal. These platforms offer a cornucopia of information and tools that aid in tracking your nutritional intake and physical activity with a few clicks and taps. Engage with these resources as companions, ones that keep your goals in sight and your progress charted.

When the body's whispers turn into a cry for sleep and rest, found wisdom waits on the pages of "Why We Sleep" by Matthew Walker.

This essential reading unveils the science behind our need for slumber and its undervalued importance in weight management and overall health.

The mindscape, as tumultuous and mysterious as the deepest oceans, can be navigated with help from texts like "The Willpower Instinct" by Kelly McGonigal. This book serves as a compass to strengthen one's mental resolve and understand the underpinnings of self-control in the pursuit of health goals.

Blending the ancient with the modern, the digital resource Headspace.com provides an oasis where meditation and mindfulness are demystified. Both newcomers and seasoned practitioners can find serenity here and fortify their mental resilience while easing stress that often coexists with weight loss endeavors.

Community and support can be paramount. Websites like SparkPeople.com foster online tribes where encouragement is but a message away. Lean on such communities as you would a friend, and offer your strength in return. It's a symbiotic relationship that can carry you through the thorniest of brambles on your journey.

The perils of misinformation are rife, yet fear not, for precision nutrition information can be found within the pages of "The China Study" by T. Colin Campbell and Thomas M. Campbell. In this work, you'll uncover connections between diet and chronic diseases and unearth dietary truths grounded in rigorous science.

Turning to the world wide web, explore sites like PrecisionNutrition.com, which marries the science of nutrition with the art of coaching. Here, knowledge is shared not just for consumption but for transformation.

For the holistic-minded seeker, "Integrative Nutrition" by Joshua Rosenthal offers a comprehensive look at nutrition that transcends the mere caloric to encompass life's myriad aspects. Pair its wisdom with that found through exploring DrWeil.com, the digital presence of a leading figure in integrative medicine, to enhance your understanding of how varied pathways to health can converge.

As our internal engines, metabolism holds curiosity and complexity, which are eloquently unpacked in Gary Taubes' work, "Why We Get Fat: And What to Do About It." Analyze the mechanisms of your body's inner workings as one would a proclamation of great importance.

Stoke the flames of your motivation at TED.com, where speeches by thought leaders can ignite the spark within. Search topics related to nutrition, wellness, and psychology, and dive into a sea of ideas worth spreading.

Finally, never underestimate the power of a well-maintained blog. Discover writers who specialize in weight loss journeys, fitness triumphs, and mental health voyage. Blogs offer an ongoing stream of fresh perspectives and can serve as a daily reminder that you belong to a wider world all striving for similar goals.

Encircled by such a wealth of resources, chart your course, and set sail on the ever-expanding ocean of knowledge. Immerse yourself in the words and wisdom of experts, and weave their teachings into the fabric of your everyday life. With each page turned and each site visited, you forge ahead on your journey to holistic health and well-being.

Recipes for Healthy Living

In the striving for vigor and vitality, we often find ourselves at the helm of the stove—where what we craft can nourish not just our bodies, but our very souls. This gregarious chapter intends to beckon you into the world where flavors and health coalesce with elegance, whispering that eating for wellness can, and indeed should, be a delightful affair. Let's embark on a culinary odyssey, offering up dishes that are as pleasing to the palate as they are conducive to a healthful existence.

These recipes are more than just combinations of ingredients—alluring as they are—they stand as testament to the fact that eating healthily does not necessitate a sacrifice of the sensual pleasures that food can offer. Each meal we partake in can be a jubilant celebration, an infusion of energy, and a step on the path to weight loss and well-being. So, whether you're a seasoned chef or a novice in the kitchen, these culinary concoctions have been devised to inspire and to fuel your wellness adventure.

A salad should not elicit sighs of dietary resignation. Instead, imagine leafy greens tossed with a vibrant array of vegetables; red and yellow peppers cut into slender strips, tomatoes bursting with ripeness, and a modest crumble of feta cheese that adds a tangy contrast. It's a symphony of color and crunch, drizzled with an olive oil and lemon vinaigrette that's both zesty and heart-healthy. A salad, yes, but one that dances on the tongue and contributes to your nutritional harmony.

To satiate and soothe, think of soups that warm the heart without weighing down the spirit. Consider a broth-based melody of seasonal vegetables, perhaps with gentle whispers of garlic and herbs for a song of flavors. Slow-simmered, such soups marry well-being with satisfaction, offering a hearty embrace without lingering too long on the waist.

Grilled dishes of fish, resplendent with omega-3 fatty acids, possess the power to transform a simple meal into an exquisite sea-bound journey. Anointed with herbs, these fillets require not the heavy hand of sauces but celebrate the richness of their oceanic origins, provided they're cooked with a light touch, respecting the delicate nature of the fare. Grilling, moreover, is a culinary art form that pays homage to the integrity of the ingredients, requiring little more than heat, a dash of seasoning, and a watchful eye.

Vegetarians, neither forgotten nor forlorn in our kitchen, can delve into the rustic charm of legumes, transformed from humble beginnings into stews and patties that boast both protein and pleasure. Grains, too, offer a vast canvas upon which to paint with bold flavors and textures: quinoa adorned with a medley of roasted vegetables, or a hearty bulgur pilaf, for instance. These too are robust paths to wellness, leaving one satiated and content.

For those who venture into the post-dinner sweet, fear not the downfall of your diligence. Desserts can still serenade your sensibilities without leading you astray. A fruit parfait layered with Greek yogurt—rich in proteins and probiotics—is not merely a concession to health, but an act of pure indulgence. It's a testament to the fact that sweetness in life need not be shunned but celebrated mindfully.

Smoothies, those harmonious blends of fruits and sometimes verdant greens, can serve as a meal replacement or a nutritional interlude, offering both refreshment and sustenance. With the correct calibration of ingredients, one can craft a potion to promote satiety, invigorate the senses, and imbue the body with vitamins, minerals, and life force.

It's of paramount importance to remember that every ingredient weaves its own narrative into the greater story of the dish. Choose whole, unprocessed foods and your meals will not only become a source of nutrients but also a celebration of natural flavors. These recipes are a tapestry of such selections, woven together to create a culinary quilt that comforts and protects our well-being.

And let's not neglect the seasonings, those humble heroes of the kitchen. They not only elevate the taste but can offer additional health benefits. Turmeric, with its golden hue and anti-inflammatory prowess; cinnamon, sweet and heartwarming, known to aid in blood sugar control; and fresh herbs, which lend their fragrance and vitality to any dish they grace. Seasonings epitomize the idea that the best prescriptions need not come from the pharmacy but can be found in our spice racks.

Make no mistake, the preparation of these recipes is as integral to their delight as the consumption. To chop and to stir—is to meditate motion. Cooking becomes a mindful practice, a time to be fully present with each slice and simmer. As one tends to ingredients with care and attention, the kitchen is transformed into a sanctuary of tranquility and nourishment.

Instructions for these recipes will be as clear as a babbling brook, easily accessible to the novice, yet still engaging enough to entice the seasoned culinary artisan. Measurements will be exact, timing precise, yet always with room for personal interpretation and improvisation, for the kitchen is nothing if not a place of personal expression.

And what of portions, you may ask? Here, too, we will be sagely specific. Moderation is the watchword, allowing you to savor each bite with the certainty that it contributes to, rather than detracts from, your overarching wellness aims.

Above all, these recipes are invitations—to explore, to taste, to experiment. They are stepping stones on your journey toward a robust life, one where healthfulness and pleasure walk hand in hand, pausing often to delight in the wonders of the world's bounty prepared at your own hands.

As you continue your exploration of mindful wellness, let this treasury of recipes serve as your culinary compass—guiding you through the thrills of new flavor landscapes and the comforting embrace of wholesome, nourishing meals. These are the recipes for a healthy life; they are the recipes for your life.

Exercise Programs and Guides

Embarking on the path to greater health and wellness through physical activity necessitates finding the right guide to light the way. Knowing which exercise programs will complement your journey best is not just about matching your workout to your current fitness level, but also intertwining it with your personal wellness goals and lifestyle. It's not about sheer rigor or relentless repetition but about discovering the routines that resonate with your body and spirit, much like finding a melody that moves you to dance.

Let us delve into a cornucopia of exercise programs that cater to your preferences, whether you fancy the solitary struggle against inertia within the confines of your home gym or the collective energy of a class pulsates with your heartbeat. You'll find solace in the fact that there isn't a singular road to fitness; but rather, a sprawling network of trails waiting to be explored by eager feet.

Indulge your curiosity in high-intensity interval training (HIIT), where the swift ebb and flow of exertion and rest not only ignites your metabolism but also infuses your schedule with efficiency. The thrill of pushing your boundaries for brief, explosive intervals juxtaposed with moments of respite can yield remarkable results, reshaping both body and spirit with purposeful quickness.

Alternatively, if the grounding practice of yoga beckons you with its promise of balance and flexibility, you'll find a diverse collection of styles and intensities. From the tranquility of Hatha, the dynamic flow of Vinyasa, to the strenuous postures of Ashtanga, one can weave mindfulness and breath through each movement, embodying a flowing meditation.

Lifting weights needn't be an intimidating pursuit of Herculean physique. Strength training can be a sculptor's tool, where resistance shapes the muscles and fortifies bone-density with every deliberate lift. Programs within this domain encourage a persistent, progressive challenge to one's own strength, always leaving room for growth and adaptation.

For those whose joy is found in the rhythmic beating of pavement beneath their feet, running programs abound, from couch-to-5k plans for novices, all the way to marathon training schedules for the seasoned runner. Each step a testament to progress, a culmination of countless resilient strides.

Let's not forget the importance of low-impact exercises for those either beginning their fitness journey or seeking gentler options. Swimming glides to the forefront, an endeavor that harnesses the resistance of water to train nearly every muscle, all the while cushioning the body from harsh impacts.

Pilates emerges as a methodology centered on mind-body synergy. Core strength, control, and precision constitute the pillars of this practice, with a vast array of exercises to suit individuals of varying abilities and aspirations. It's a pilgrimage to the heart of your physical center, your core, teaching poise and balance.

Then there are the hybrid systems, fusion workouts like barre, which intertwine the discipline of ballet with the alignment of yoga and the strength elements of Pilates. There's something invigorating about finding balance within these combinations, much like crafting a new language from familiar words.

For those enchanted by rhythm and the joy of collective motion, dance-based fitness classes such as Zumba and Hip-Hop workouts offer a blend of infectious music and choreographed movements that sculpt the body while freeing the soul. It's a celebration of movement, each gyration an echo of wellness.

Circuit training, too, must be mentioned: a buffet of exercises that gives the whole body a taste of exertion. It's an adventure around various stations where muscles meet diverse challenges, ensuring a comprehensive cut of wellness served with dynamic rest.

Bodyweight programs demonstrate that one's own weight provides enough resistance to forge strength and endurance. With no need for equipment, these programs empower you to claim your fitness anytime, anywhere – your body as both the anvil and the hammer in this craft of physical betterment.

Let's not neglect the digital landscape's offerings; a plethora of apps and online platforms are at your fingertips, each boasting an array of workouts designed by seasoned professionals and tailored to a smorgasbord of goals and preferences.

Athletes or those with spirited competitive streaks can leap into sport-specific training routines, refining the skills and building the physical prowess necessary to excel in their chosen domain. Each drill is a step closer to mastery, turning the sport itself into an avenue for fitness.

Ultimately, the guides and programs are as diverse as the individuals who undertake them. It is up to you to elect your pathway and embrace the journey it unfolds. Regardless of the program you choose, the focus remains unified; to animate your life with vigor and purpose, to challenge and to cherish every exertion, to embark upon a voyage that not only transforms the body but elevates the spirit. Here, in these curated guides, you'll find the blueprints for your corporeal temple, the drafts for your well-being destiny.

As we close this section, it is imperative to acknowledge that the right exercise program is not set in stone but is a dynamic part of your overall life journey. Adaptability, patience, and an enduring curiosity will be your steadfast companions, together sculpting the silhouette of your future self.